1. FOREWORD

Welcome to edition 36 of
Medicines, Ethics and Practice (MEP).

Reflecting the evolution of the Royal Pharmaceutical Society into the professional body for pharmacists on 27 September 2010, and the transfer of regulatory roles to the General Pharmaceutical Council, the MEP continues to evolve.

This professional guide for pharmacists has been designed as an underpinning document to help pharmacists practise confidently and professionally. It embeds professionalism and professional judgment at the heart of the decision-making process.

This continues the MEP's tradition of providing information and guidance on legislation affecting pharmacy practice; supporting day-to-day practice rather than simply highlighting pharmacists' statutory obligations.

The MEP is written by the RPS Support team a small team of pharmacists and advisors from different pharmacy sectors. The team works in collaboration with specialist colleagues within the professional body and external experts within the profession and produces a range of guidance materials to support members in their day-to-day practice. It also provides online support at **www.rpharms.com**, by telephone on 0845 257 2570 or 0207 572 2737, or by email at support@rpharms.com.

One free copy of the MEP is distributed to all pharmacist members and associate members. All members, including student members benefit from free online access and discounted purchase prices. Copies of MEP are available for

DISCLAIMER

This publication is intended as a guide and may not always include all information relating to its subject matter. You should interpret all information and advice in light of your own professional knowledge and all relevant pharmacy and healthcare literature and guidelines. Nothing in this publication constitutes legal advice and cannot be relied upon as such. Whilst care has been taken to ensure the accuracy of content RPSGB excludes to the fullest extent permissible by law any liability whether in contract, tort or otherwise arising from your reliance on any information or advice.

general purchase at a cost of £49.99 and are available from the Pharmaceutical Press website at **www.pharmpress.com** or by telephone from Pharmaceutical Press c/o Macmillan on Tel: 0203 318 3141

We welcome comments and feedback; these can be sent to us using the contact details above or by post to RPS Support, Royal Pharmaceutical Society 1 Lambeth High Street, London SE1 7JN.

CONTENTS

CONTENTS

APPENDICES

2. CORE CONCEPTS AND SKILLS

2.1 Professionalism and professional judgment

It is important to recognise that pharmacy is not just any occupation; it is a profession and pharmacists are professionals who exercise professionalism and professional judgment on a day-to-day basis.

The concepts of a 'profession', a 'professional' and 'professionalism' are not rigidly defined. However these are concepts that are important for any pharmacist.

A profession can be described as:

■ An occupation that is recognised by the public as a profession

■ An occupation for which there is a recognised representative professional body

■ An occupation that benefits from professional standards and codes of conduct

■ An occupation that is regulated to ensure the maintenance of standards and codes of conduct

A professional can be described as:

■ A member of a profession

■ A member of a professional body

■ An individual who:

● behaves and acts professionally

● exercises professionalism and professional judgment, and

● has professional values, attitudes and behaviours

Professionalism

Pharmacy professionalism can be defined as a set of values, behaviours and relationships that underpin the trust the public has in pharmacists. Examples of these are:

■ Altruism

■ Appropriate accountability

■ Compassion

■ Duty

■ Excellence and continuous improvement

■ Honour and integrity

■ Professional judgment

■ Respect for other patients, colleagues and other healthcare professionals

■ Working in partnership with patients, doctors and the wider healthcare team in the patient's/public's best interest

Many of these values, attitudes and behaviours are also reflected in the mandatory GPhC standards for conduct, ethics and performance (see Appendix 1).

Professional judgment

Professional judgment can be described as the use of accumulated knowledge and experience, as well as critical reasoning, to make an informed professional decision – often to solve or ameliorate a problem presented by, or in relation to, a patient; or policies and procedures affecting patients. It takes into account the law, ethical considerations, relevant standards and all other relevant factors related to the surrounding circumstances. Furthermore, it will resonate with the core values, attitudes and behavioural indicators of professionalism.

How do I exercise professional judgment?

Many pharmacists exercise their professional judgment instinctively but it may be helpful to break the process down into smaller steps:

1. Identify the ethical dilemma or professional issue
2. Gather all relevant information and research the problem – i.e. obtain relevant:
   - facts
   - knowledge
   - laws
   - standards
   - good practice guidance
   - advice from support services, head office, line managers or colleagues
3. Identify the possible options
4. Weigh up the benefits, risks, advantages and disadvantages of each option
5. Choose an option, ensuring that you can justify your decision based upon the above points
6. Where appropriate, make a record of the decision-making process and your reasons leading to a particular course of action. It may be appropriate to make this record in the patient's medical record, the back of the prescription register or an interventions record book. This is important as evidence of the thought processes leading to a decision.

It is entirely possible for two different pharmacists, faced with the same facts and circumstances, to choose two different courses of action. That is the nature of a finely balanced ethical dilemma. Both options could be justifiable and legitimate choices for a significant proportion of pharmacists if faced with the same dilemma.

The process of making a professional judgment is underpinned by knowledge. The following chapters of the MEP provide information on the core knowledge required by pharmacists in their day-to-day practice.

REFERENCES AND FURTHER READING

American Board of Internal Medicine. *Project Professionalism* (7th printing). Philadelphia: the board; 2001.

Appelbe G, Wingfield J. *Dale and Appelbe's Pharmacy Law and Ethics.* London: Pharmaceutical Press; 2009.

Elvey R, Lewis P, Schafheutle E, Willis S, Harrison S, Hassel K *Patient-centred professionalism among newly registered pharmacists* 2011. **www.pprt.org.uk**; select the publications tab.

Pharmacy Law and Ethics Association (PLEA) – an independent group and a partner of the Royal Pharmaceutical Society of persons interested in pharmacy, law and ethics. The PLEA virtual network is available to PLEA subscribers on the RPS website (**www.rpharms.com**).

Royal College of Physicians working party. *Doctors in society: Medical professionalism in a changing world.* London: the college; 2005.

Schafheutle E, Hassell K, Ashcroft D, et al. *Professionalism in pharmacy education.* 2010. **www.pprt.org.uk**; select the publications tab.

Wingfield J, Badcott D. *Pharmacy Ethics and Decision Making.* London: Pharmaceutical Press; 2007.

2.2 Clinical check

One of the key skills of a pharmacist when supplying medicines to patients is to perform a fundamental clinical assessment or clinical check of the medicine to be supplied. Clinical checks involve identifying potential pharmacotherapeutic problems by collating and evaluating all relevant information, including patient characteristics, disease states, medication regimen and, where possible, laboratory results.

Importantly it is not a mere dose and interaction check, or a simple tick box exercise but rather a complex skill which will often require interaction with patients and healthcare professionals. A clinical check is underpinned by knowledge of human pathophysiology as well as medicines (pharmacokinetics, pharmacology, pharmaceutics, pharmacognosy) coupled with clinical experience and the rational application of professional judgment. It is a key part of clinical pharmacy contributing to patient safety and public health.

Recent evidence-based studies including EQUIP by Dornan et al which looked at causes of prescribing errors and the PINCER trial by Avery et al which looked at pharmacist-led technology enabled interventions, highlight the benefit of the clinical input by pharmacists.

By using a structured, logical approach to clinically check, pharmacists can balance the risks and benefits of a prescribed medicine regimen and, in doing so, improve the medicine's safety and effectiveness.

The areas that pharmacists need to consider when undertaking a clinical check include:

■ Patient characteristics

■ Medication regimen

■ How treatment will be administered and monitored

OBTAINING INFORMATION

The sources for obtaining information, and the level of detail available, will vary depending on the pharmacy setting. It may not always be practicable to obtain all the information needed and, sometimes, decisions will need to be made on limited information.

In primary care, you may be able to obtain information from:

■ The prescription

■ The patient, patient's representative or carer

■ The patient's GP or other healthcare professionals involved in the patient's care

■ The patient's medication record

■ Other patient medical records where available (e.g. in Scotland – access to the Emergency Care Summary; in a prison – access to medical records)

In secondary care, additional sources of information available would include other healthcare professionals involved in the patient's care (e.g. dieticians, microbiologists and physiotherapists), medical and nursing care notes, additional ward charts and laboratory results.

Patient characteristics

Factors relating to patient characteristics that should be considered during a clinical check include:

- **PATIENT TYPE** – establish whether the patient falls into a group where treatment is contraindicated or cautioned. Specific groups of patients to be aware of include:
  - children
  - women who are pregnant or breastfeeding
  - the elderly
  - certain ethnic groups – a patient's ethnic origin can affect the choice of medicine or dose (e.g. the initial and maximum dose of rosuvastatin is lower for patients of Asian origin)

  (For some medicines, the gender of the patient should be considered. For example, finasteride is contraindicated for women.)

- **CO-MORBIDITIES** – patient co-morbidities, such as renal or hepatic impairment or heart failure, can exclude the use of a particular treatment or necessitate dose adjustments

- **PATIENT INTOLERANCES AND PREFERENCES** – other patient factors that can affect the choice of treatment include known medication adverse events (e.g. allergies), dietary intolerances (e.g. to lactose-containing products), patient preferences (e.g. vegan patients may refuse products of porcine origin), religious beliefs, and patients knowledge and understanding of medicines and why they are being taken (patient beliefs about medicines)

Medication regimen factors

Aspects of the prescribed medication regimen that should be considered during a clinical check include:

- **INDICATION** – ascertain the indication for treatment to check whether the medicine prescribed is appropriate for the indication and compatible with recommended guidelines

- **CHANGES IN REGULAR TREATMENT** – where there are changes in regular therapy (e.g. strength or dose), pharmacists should confirm that these are intentional

- **DOSE, FREQUENCY AND STRENGTH** – pharmacists should check that the dose, frequency and strength of the prescribed medicine are appropriate – having considered the patient's age, renal and hepatic function, weight (and surface area where appropriate), co-morbidities, concomitant drug treatments and lifestyle pattern

- **THE DOSING OF THE FORMULATION** – check that, for the formulation prescribed, the dose and frequency are appropriate

- **DRUG COMPATIBILITY** – regular and new therapies should be evaluated for any clinically significant interactions, duplications and antagonistic activity

- **MONITORING REQUIREMENTS** – for medicines that require monitoring, pharmacists should check for the latest test results and ascertain whether any dose adjustments are required

Administration and monitoring

Aspects relating to the administration and monitoring of a medicine that should be considered during a clinical check include:

- **THE ROUTE OF ADMINISTRATION** – check whether the prescribed route of administration is suitable for the patient and whether a preparation is available for that route. Also, check for compatibility issues that may arise from administering via that route (e.g. due to co-administration of food or other medicines). For example, phenytoin can interact with enteral feeds so administration via an enteral feeding tube would need to be managed accordingly

- **THE NEED FOR ADMINISTRATION AIDS** – check whether any adherence aids required by the patient are available. For example, spacer devices, eye drop devices, Braille or large type or pictogram labels, additional information sheets or verbal information

Record Keeping

Record keeping is important for continuity of care, evidence of the benefit of pharmacy input and improving patient care and pharmacists should make a record of significant clinical checks, and interventions made. This should include details of discussions and agreed decisions with other healthcare professionals. Depending upon the circumstances it may be appropriate to make this record in the patient's medical record, an interventions record book, hand-over record book or prescription register.

REFERENCES AND FURTHER READING

British National Formulary (**www.bnf.org**)

British National Formulary for Children (**www.bnfc.org**)

Clinical Pharmacist (**www.pjonline.com/clinical-pharmacist**)

Stephens M. *Hospital Pharmacy* (2nd edition). London: Pharmaceutical Press; 2011.

Wright J, Gray A, Goodey V. *Clinical Pharmacy Pocket Companion.* London: Pharmaceutical Press; 2006.

RPS Support. Clinical check quick reference guide. 2011. (**www.rpharms.com**)

Dornan T, Ashcroft D, Heathfield H, Lewis P, Miles J, Taylor D, et al. *An in depth investigation into causes of prescribing errors by foundation trainees in relation to their medical education. EQUIP Study.* London: General Medical Council 2009.

Avery AJ, Rodgers S, Cantrill JA, Armstrong S, Cresswell K, Eden M, et al. *Pharmacist-led information technology-enabled intervention for reducing medication errors: Multi-centre cluster randomised controlled trial and cost-effectiveness analysis (PINCER Trial).* The Lancet. 2012.

2.3 Taking medication histories

An accurate medication history provides a foundation for assessing the appropriateness of a patient's current medicines and directing future treatment choices. It can prevent medication errors and, during the process of obtaining a history, allows other pharmaceutical issues (such as poor- or non-adherence) to be identified. It is important, as part of a pharmacist's clinical role, that any medication histories taken are accurate to help ensure a patient's current and future therapy is safe and effective.

Sources of information

Sources of information that may be used when taking a medication history include:

1. Patient or patient's representative
2. Patient's medicines
3. Repeat prescriptions
4. GP referral letters
5. The patient's GP surgery
6. Hospital discharge summaries or outpatient appointment notes
7. Community pharmacy patient medication records
8. Care home records
9. Drug treatment centre records
10. Other healthcare professionals and specialist clinics
11. Patient medical records where available (e.g. in prisons or the Emergency Care Summary in Scotland)

GENERAL TIPS FOR OBTAINING A MEDICATION HISTORY

- Explain to the patient why the history is being taken

- Use a balance of open-ended questions (e.g. what, how, why, when) with closed questions (i.e. those requiring yes/no answers)

- Avoid jargon – keep it simple

- Clarify vague responses with further questioning or by using other sources of information

- Keep the patient at ease

Key points

ARE THE SOURCES YOU USE UP-TO-DATE? Aim to use the most complete, reliable and up-to-date source(s) of information.

CROSS-CHECK ADHERENCE Medication histories should be cross-checked against different sources and confirmed with the patient or patient's representative. The medicines they are actually taking, and how they are taking them, may differ from written documentation (e.g. the prescribing record held by the patient's GP).

NON-DAILY MEDICINES Remember to ask patients whether they take any medicines 'when required' (e.g. reliever inhalers), or on certain days of the week. Also remember to ask about the sorts of formulations that might be forgotten (e.g. nasal sprays, eye or ear drops, ointments, depot injections, patches, etc). Patients may also need prompting to remember medicines such as oral contraceptives and hormone replacement therapy.

HISTORICAL MEDICINES The medication history should not be restricted to current therapies but should include any recently stopped or changed medicines.

SELF-SELECTED MEDICINES Include any medicinal product that the patient is taking – whether prescribed or not – and do not restrict the medication history to medicines obtained on prescription. Over-the-counter (OTC) medicines, herbal products, vitamins, dietary supplements, recreational drugs (e.g. alcohol and tobacco) and remedies purchased over the internet should also be included.

What information should I obtain when taking a medication history?

For each medicine, the following should be determined:

- Generic name of the drug
- Brand name of the drug, where appropriate (for example, where bioavailability variations between brands can have clinical consequences, such as lithium therapy)
- Dose – both the prescribed dose and the actual dose the patient is taking (NB: This may best be described to the patient as a quantity of tablets rather than as milligrams of active ingredient)
- Strength of the medicine taken
- Formulation used (e.g. phenytoin – 100mg as a liquid does not deliver the same dose as a 100mg tablet)
- Route of administration (this could be an unlicensed route – e.g. ciprofloxacin eye drops for the ear)
- Frequency of administration – this should include the time of administration for certain medicines (e.g. levodopa)
- Length of therapy, if appropriate (e.g. for antibiotics)
- Administration device and brand for injectables (e.g. insulin)
- Day or date of administration for medicines taken on specific days of the week or month

In addition, for medicines requiring a variable dosing regimen (e.g. warfarin), details of the daily regimen, target level and monitoring arrangements should be ascertained. Ask to see any patient monitoring booklets where applicable (e.g. insulin passport, methotrexate booklet, oral anticoagulant booklet).

FURTHER READING

Stephens M. *Hospital Pharmacy* (2nd edition). London: Pharmaceutical Press; 2011.

RPS Support. *Medication history – quick reference guide.* 2011. (**www.rpharms.com**)

National Institute for Health and Clinical Excellence *Technical patient safety solutions for medicines reconciliation on admission of adults to hospital.* December 2007. (**www.nice.org.uk**)

2.4 Counselling patients

An important key role of a pharmacist is to be able to counsel patients ensuring that they understand their medicines, the role that their medicines play in maintaining their well-being, empowering patients to use them safely and effectively. Counselling involves being able to build a rapport with the patient, good communication skills, empathy, being able to put the patient at ease, and being able to confer an understanding and belief that the health of the patient is important to the pharmacist.

Involving and engaging the patient in the counselling process will improve concordance.

Opportunities for counselling

Medication counselling opportunities should not be limited to when a supply of newly prescribed medicines is made, and almost any interaction with the patient can be used as an opportunity to initiate medication counselling. A simple question asking 'How are you getting on with your medicines' can often be a successful engaging starting point. Illustrative examples of opportunities for counselling include:

- Point of sale for over-the-counter medicines
- Medicines Use Reviews (England and Wales)
- Diagnostic testing and screening
- Patient group directions
- Minor ailment schemes
- Whilst taking medication history
- During a hospital stay
- Point of discharge
- Outpatient clinics
- When a change has been made to a current medicine
- Point of a supply of a regular prescription

Advice for better counselling

- Try to understand the level of existing knowledge, understanding and concerns the patient has regarding their medicines. Consider any misunderstandings which could be a barrier to adherence. Explore what the patient has already been told about their medicines, whether there are any concerns, and what the patient's expectations are

- Ensure you are familiar with the medicine you will be providing counselling on and any additional counselling relevant to that medicine. If in doubt, take time to review and re-familiarise yourself with the medicine. For example – look out for interactions with other medicines, food, or supplements, or medicines with common or significant side effects, complex administration regimens, special storage requirements, or narrow therapeutic index. Check standard references (e.g. BNF or national guidelines for additional counselling information)

- Aim for a structured approach and tailor the language and level of detail used to the patient. The type of counselling you provide will depend upon both patient characteristics and the medicines which are taken. As an illustration the needs of patients with language or literacy problems or patients with new medication will more often require more counselling

- Where appropriate use medication counselling aids such as pictograms and medication cards

- Respect patient privacy and ensure that confidentiality is protected

- Ensure that the process is a two-way interactive process and not simply a list of facts about medicines. There should be opportunities for questions and discussion

When counselling, you should as a minimum consider providing the following information:

- What is the medicine and why has it been prescribed? How does it impact upon the medical condition and how does it alleviate the symptoms? e.g. *This is a blood pressure medicine which is used to lower your blood pressure to normal levels which will help prevent further complications*

- How and when to take the medicine

- How much to take and what to expect e.g. antibiotics need to be taken regularly and the course completed even after symptoms subside

- What to do if the patient misses a dose

- What are the likely side effects and how to manage them

- If applicable, any lifestyle or dietary changes that need to be made or that can affect the treatment

■ Additional information relating to storage requirements, expiry dates, disposal and monitoring requirements can also be included where appropriate

■ Check patient understanding of the counselling provided by asking the patient to describe back to you the key information you have provided

FURTHER RESOURCES

CPPE. *Confidence in consultation skills* (a workshop for pharmacists). (**www.cppe.ac.uk**)

NICE guidance Medicines adherence: Involving patients in decisions about prescribed medicines and supporting adherence (**www.nice.org.uk**)

RPS Support. Medicines adherence (NICE implementation) guidance for pharmacists. (**www.rpharms.com**)

Hugman, Bruce *Healthcare Communication* (1st edition). London. Pharmaceutical Press; 2009

RPS Support. Counselling patients – quick reference guide (**www.rpharms.com**)

GP-training.net. Patient counselling resources and concise information regarding the Cambridge-Calgary model for patient counselling. (**www.gp-training.net**)

2.5 Just culture

A *just culture* is a culture which is based upon fairness and is achieved when attitudes, behaviour and practices are in accordance with what is fair and right.

It differs from a *punitive culture* which is a culture based upon punishment but which also stifles learning and reporting of concerns.

It also differs from a *no-blame culture* which is based on the concept of never assigning blame but suffers from lack of accountability.

Why is it needed?

A *just culture* makes people and patients safer compared with the alternative *punitive* culture or *no-blame* culture. It achieves this by promoting fairer accountability and a necessary learning culture.

Upon application to the provision of healthcare and pharmacy services, this entails being able to learn from mistakes or incidents, to be able to share lessons learnt (throughout the profession where appropriate) and to use this shared learning to reduce the likelihood of similar mistakes and incidents from happening again, which is a vital component contributing to making patients safer.

When a mistake or incident occurs, we all want assurances that actions are being taken so that it will *never happen again* and that there will be fair accountability. Whilst a *just culture* cannot guarantee mistakes or incidents will not re-occur it can and does help to prevent them from happening in the first place.

Does it already exist?

In some places Yes.

Just culture principles may be incorporated in attitudes, behaviours, systems, standards, policies, regulations and legislation and may already be compatible with the culture of some organisations.

In places where it doesn't exist, we must all work towards embedding a *just culture*.

Where it already exists, this should be celebrated and supported to enable continued commitment to *just culture* principles.

How do we collectively achieve a *just culture*?

The journey to achieving a *just culture* requires the embedding of *just culture* principles into attitudes, behaviours, practices and the design of legislation, regulations, standards, policies and systems.

It will require commitment by **all** stakeholders (Government bodies, regulatory bodies, Royal Pharmaceutical Society, academic institutions, trade associations, indemnity providers, unions, NHS and private employers, pharmacists and patient groups) to apply *just culture* principles on a daily basis, and through all activities and all interfaces with other stakeholders. It is a continuous evolving project and may take years or decades to achieve, but one to which the Royal Pharmaceutical Society and others are committed.

For the Royal Pharmaceutical Society, it means applying *just culture* principles to all that we do, encouraging engagement of all other stakeholders with the *just culture* philosophy and viewing all of our outputs and interactions with other stakeholders through a prism of *just culture*. For example, whenever we respond to a new initiative, we must consider if it impacts upon a *just culture*.

Just culture and patient safety incidents

Patient safety can be improved by the reporting of concerns and learning from these reports. The reporting of concerns will only take place if individuals feel they will not be victimised and that it is 'safe' to report these concerns. To provide assurance and confidence, everybody needs to know where they stand.

The airline industry has been embedding *just culture* principles into its practices for decades to improve safety. Adapting from what they have learnt, together with consideration of similar workstreams within the NHS, we believe in the following *just culture* principles for patient safety incidents:

1. Patient safety is paramount

2. Deliberate harm and unacceptable risk impacting on patient safety must not be tolerated

3. Patient safety is maintained by raising concerns and learning from incidents to improve systems, standards, policies, legislation and people

4. To ensure that concerns will be raised and learning from incidents occurs, individual accountability must always be fair and proportionate, and viewed in the context of root cause, system deficiencies, mitigating circumstances and the entirety of contributing factors (*i.e. the whole picture*)

The NHS has developed an incident decision tree based upon the work of Professor James Reason, an expert on patient safety. This decision-making tool embodies *just culture* principles and uses a series of tests to decide on the appropriate course of action following an incident.

FURTHER READING

Decker S, *Just Culture: Balancing Safety and Accountability* Ashgate 2007

Meadows S, Baker K, Butler J. *The incident decision tree: guidelines for action following patient safety incidents.* In: **Henriksen K, Battles JB, Marks ES, et al., editors.** *Advances in Patient Safety: From Research to Implementation* (Volume 4: Programs, Tools, and Products). Rockville (MD): Agency for Healthcare Research and Quality (US); February 2005

GPhC, *Guidance on raising concerns* (February 2012) (**www.pharmacyregulation.org**) (see also Appendix 6)

RPS. *Raising concerns, whistle blowing and speaking up safely in Pharmacy* (September 2011) (**www.rpharms.com**)

RPS. *8 core principles for community pharmacy whistle blowing policies and procedures* (September 2011) (**www.rpharms.com**)

CORE CONCEPTS AND SKILLS

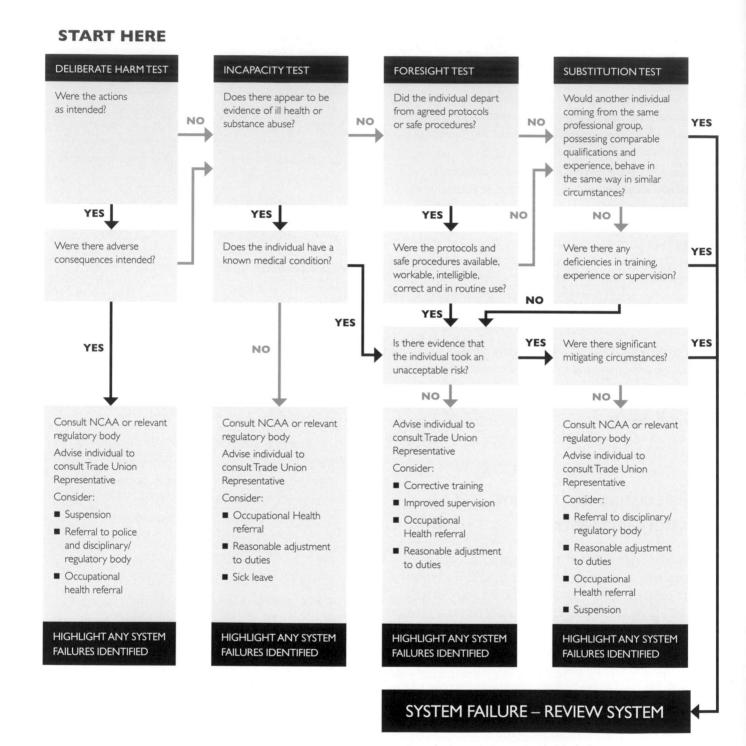

DELIBERATE HARM TEST

Were the actions as intended?

YES ↓

Were there adverse consequences intended?

YES ↓

Consult NCAA or relevant regulatory body

Advise individual to consult Trade Union Representative

Consider:
- Suspension
- Referral to police and disciplinary/ regulatory body
- Occupational health referral

HIGHLIGHT ANY SYSTEM FAILURES IDENTIFIED

NO →

INCAPACITY TEST

Does there appear to be evidence of ill health or substance abuse?

YES ↓

Does the individual have a known medical condition?

NO ↓

Consult NCAA or relevant regulatory body

Advise individual to consult Trade Union Representative

Consider:
- Occupational Health referral
- Reasonable adjustment to duties
- Sick leave

HIGHLIGHT ANY SYSTEM FAILURES IDENTIFIED

NO →

FORESIGHT TEST

Did the individual depart from agreed protocols or safe procedures?

YES ↓

Were the protocols and safe procedures available, workable, intelligible, correct and in routine use?

YES ↓

Is there evidence that the individual took an unacceptable risk?

NO ↓

Advise individual to consult Trade Union Representative

Consider:
- Corrective training
- Improved supervision
- Occupational Health referral
- Reasonable adjustment to duties

HIGHLIGHT ANY SYSTEM FAILURES IDENTIFIED

NO →

SUBSTITUTION TEST

Would another individual coming from the same professional group, possessing comparable qualifications and experience, behave in the same way in similar circumstances?

NO → (from Foresight)

NO ↓

Were there any deficiencies in training, experience or supervision?

NO ↓

YES → Were there significant mitigating circumstances?

NO ↓

Consult NCAA or relevant regulatory body

Advise individual to consult Trade Union Representative

Consider:
- Referral to disciplinary/ regulatory body
- Reasonable adjustment to duties
- Occupational Health referral
- Suspension

HIGHLIGHT ANY SYSTEM FAILURES IDENTIFIED

YES (Substitution Test)
YES (deficiencies in training)
YES (significant mitigating circumstances)

SYSTEM FAILURE – REVIEW SYSTEM

DIAGRAM 1: REPRODUCTION OF THE NHS INCIDENT DECISION TREE

We have included the NHS incident decision tree which is subject to crown copyright and reproduced under the terms of the Open Government Licence as an illustration of a process which is fair and balances learning and accountability.

NCAA stands for National Clinical Assessment Authority and became part of the National Clinical Assessment Service (NCAS).

2.6 Professional empowerment

Professional empowerment is about enabling professionalism.

At an individual level for pharmacists and future pharmacists, it is about the development of knowledge; development of skills, experience and confidence; and the cultivation of professional values and behaviours which collectively imbue the pharmacist with authority, empowering and enabling professionalism.

At a wider level it is about creating an environment around an individual which enables all of the above.

Professional training starts at university and is enhanced with pre-registration training by learning, pre-registration tutors and training programmes. In professional practice it is self-cultivated through *continuing professional development (CPD)* (see section 2.7) and continuing education and supported by pharmacy organisations through training programmes and events;

The Royal Pharmaceutical Society contributes to creating empowerment through guidance, standards, news and alerts; through webinars and our mentoring programme; through our leadership competency framework; through influencing policy and embedding and nurturing *just culture* (see section 2.5).

Employers play a key role by providing structured training resources and events; conferences; opportunity and time for CPD; support from the superintendent or office of the superintendent; company alerts and updates; developing and implementing the right organisation culture which enables professional empowerment.

Other pharmacy organisations, stakeholders and training providers are also integral to enabling professionalism through training and enabling the right environment for professionalism to flourish, including through *just culture*.

> ## FURTHER RESOURCES
>
> **RPS.** *Leadership competency framework for pharmacy professionals.* (**www.rpharms.com**)
>
> **RPS.** *Reducing workplace pressure through professional empowerment* (July 2011) (**www.rpharms.com**)

2.7 Continuing professional development

Pharmacists are committed to remaining competent to practise and to deliver high-quality care to patients by continually expanding their knowledge, skills and attributes throughout their working lives. Continuing professional development (CPD) plays an integral role in their careers by enhancing confidence and credibility.

By reflecting on your learning, you can identify gaps within your knowledge, skills and experience. This also allows you to identify training activities that will improve the way you deal with difficult circumstances in the future.

There is a statutory requirement for you to record your CPD. The General Pharmaceutical Council has published standards for CPD (see Appendix 3) and pharmacists are required to meet them. An annual declaration of compliance with the requirements for CPD is obligatory for registration with the GPhC.

The current GPhC standards state that registrants must make a minimum of nine CPD entries per registration year

with three of these starting at the reflection phase of the CPD cycle. These must also be relevant to the safe and effective practice of pharmacy and your own scope of practice, including any annotations for specialisations (e.g. QP, Ipresc) and the environment in which they practise. 'Scope of practice' relates to the area or areas in which a registrant practises or intends to practise. The GPhC has defined specific criteria for reviewing CPD records and for good recording practice as part of its framework for CPD.

The GPhC CPD review process follows a rotational calling for records at least once every five years (or more frequently if required). Once records have been reviewed, feedback is generated electronically in the form of an executive summary and a main report.

The GPhC specifies that all entries in your CPD record submitted to them for review should follow the CPD cycle as shown in Diagram 2. The cycle consists of a four-phased learning process: reflection, planning, action and evaluation.

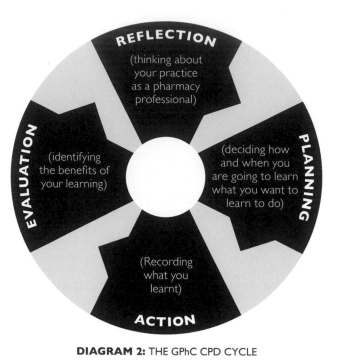

DIAGRAM 2: THE GPhC CPD CYCLE

Learning must also be recorded using a GPhC-approved CPD recording format. For most registrants, this will be an online CPD account. An approved paper recording format is also available from the GPhC.

A CPD entry may start at **reflection** if, from the outset, learning needs are identified and specific objectives can be set. This can be done through self assessment, staff appraisal, a personal development plan (PDP), peer review or through feedback received from others. For those who do not have a PDP, the GPhC online recording system has an inbuilt PDP template that can be used instead. GPhC requires that at least three CPD entries completed each year start at reflection.

Entries can also start at the **planning** phase of the CPD cycle. During this phase, the various options available to achieve specified learning objectives are considered. It is important to select one (or more) of the options that are appropriate to your scope of practice from those listed. A time frame for completing this learning should also be considered along with the advantages and disadvantages of undertaking this learning and its importance to you, users of your services and products, colleagues and your organisation.

Action is the interesting phase of the CPD cycle when the learning takes place. CPD entries can start at action if they result from unplanned learning. In the action section of a CPD entry, the activity undertaken to acquire new learning should be recorded, along with what was learned and when it was completed.

Evaluation comes at the end of the learning cycle when you assess whether you have achieved your learning objectives and, if so, how this learning may be applied and how it will benefit your practice. Application of learning may be recorded in the past, present or future tenses with clear benefits to practice, patients or the public documented. Where learning objectives are only partially met or not met at all, the required next steps should be recorded. In addition, resources might need to be allocated to complete the CPD cycle or to start a new cycle.

The GPhC guidance on CPD standards state that registrants should maintain a personal learning portfolio that will be the main source of evidence for their CPD. Since registrants are likely to learn more than the statutory requirement, they are encouraged to make more than nine entries per year in their CPD record. When a record is called for review by the GPhC, the registrant can select nine completed entries per registration year – at least three of which should start at reflection. The GPhC advises that registrants reflect on their practice at least monthly.

Opportunities for CPD

Working life presents numerous learning opportunities throughout your career. Examples include:

1. **WORK-BASED LEARNING** – for example, when a new product or technique is introduced, when undertaking work shadowing, when asked to review a protocol, when performing a quality assessment, audit or review of a critical incident or when asked to discuss your work with your manager, a peer or another professional.

2. **SELF-DIRECTED LEARNING** – this can include reading, e-learning, accessing articles from *The Pharmaceutical Journal*, writing reports, undertaking research projects or attending workshops.

3. **FORMAL LEARNING** – attending courses or study days constitute continuing education and can increase your knowledge base, which can yield a CPD entry.

4. **PROFESSIONAL ACTIVITY** – this includes participating in specialist groups, giving lectures and presentations, coaching/mentoring or performing roles for your local practice forum (LPF).

All learning that is relevant to your scope of practice, irrespective of whether or not it involved patient-facing experiences, can lead to CPD entries in your record.

How RPS can support you with CPD

CPD is important to our members and we have an ever-growing professional development and support service portfolio to assist you. You can fulfil your statutory requirements for CPD and progress beyond your minimum needs by utilising our services, which aim to empower you to take ownership of your professional development and accomplish your professional aspirations.

We deliver CPD support services through four interfaces:

- Dedicated CPD resources are available via the Royal Pharmaceutical Society website (**www.rpharms.com**), including pre-recorded CPD webinars, FAQs, hints and tips, guides and sector-specific case studies

- Assistance is available through the RPS Support team by telephone, email or online web form. The RPS Support team is available on 0845 257 2570 or **support@rpharms.com**

- LPFs deliver regular events, surgeries, workshops, peer reviews and presentations that provide support for CPD and career development, as well as networking opportunities in your local area

- Virtual network opportunities enable you to access our dedicated member CPD online group (and other specialist groups) so that you may share your personal CPD experiences and clarify any concerns relating to your learning activities. Information is available on specific CPD events across all sectors of practice through the RPS events calendar, CPD online group and the LPF virtual networks

If you are intending to return to practice, or thinking about changing your sector of practice, the Royal Pharmaceutical Society will support you in acquiring confidence and competence to undertake your new roles and responsibilities. For some, this could mean spending time in clinical practice areas or working in a community pharmacy. For others, it could mean drawing on your previous professional skills in other roles, undertaking further research or carrying out specific studies. In your preparation, you may wish to consider the following within the context of your CPD learning portfolio:

- Critical reflection of your intended practice area(s) by relating them to relevant competencies

- Analysis of your learning needs to formulate a developmental plan to meet these needs

- Reflection on your past learning and development in order to decide how you intend to demonstrate your ability to meet the GPhC standards for CPD

The Royal Pharmaceutical Society can also help you access mentors from the profession via the online mentoring database.

Our strategy embeds a vision for you, as a pharmacist, to continually develop your practice in a way that meets your needs and learning styles, and fulfils your statutory CPD requirements. We are here to help and support you in understanding what CPD is and what you need to record, and to enhance your knowledge and skills so that you are an expert in your sector of practice and your working life.

CORE CONCEPTS AND SKILLS

FURTHER READING

RPS. *Continuing professional development.* (**www.rpharms.com**; select the Development tab)

GPhC. *Standards for continuing professional development.* September 2010. (**www.pharmacyregulation.org**)

GPhC. *CPD Framework.* July 2011. (**www.pharmacyregulation.org**)

GPhC. *Plan and record.* (**www.pharmacyregulation.org**)

RPS Support. *CPD services toolkit.* December 2010. Royal Pharmaceutical Society website (**www.rpharms.com**; select the Development tab)

Webinars run by the Royal Pharmaceutical Society can be found at (**www.rpharms.com/events/webinars.asp**)

Chartered Institute of Personnel and Development. *Benefits of CPD.* (**www.cipd.co.uk**)

Department of Health. *A first class service: Quality in the new NHS.* July 1998. (**www.dh.gov.uk**)

3. UNDERPINNING KNOWLEDGE – LEGISLATION AND PROFESSIONAL ISSUES

3.1 CLASSIFICATION OF MEDICINES

3.2 PROFESSIONAL AND LEGAL ISSUES: PHARMACY MEDICINES

3.3 PROFESSIONAL AND LEGAL ISSUES: PRESCRIPTION-ONLY MEDICINES

3.4 WHOLESALE DEALING

3.5 ADDITIONAL LEGAL AND PROFESSIONAL ISSUES

3.6 VETERINARY MEDICINES

3.7 CONTROLLED DRUGS

The exercise of professional judgment by a pharmacist is underpinned by relevant knowledge. Components of this knowledge are an awareness of pharmacy legislation, professional standards and good practice.

This resource is not intended to be a complete repository of pharmacy legislation and aims instead to provide a practical resource, professional guide and digest to the most relevant aspects of pharmacy legislation.

At the time of writing MEP 36, the Medicines Act consolidation and review process was ongoing and due to be completed prior to the publication of MEP 36. The result of this will be a major consolidation of medicines legislation as the Human Medicines Regulations 2012. It is our intention to include more detail and references to specific sections of the Human Medicines Regulations in further editions of Medicines, Ethics and Practice where appropriate.

3.1 Classification of medicines

Pharmacists deal with three classes of medicinal products for humans under medicines legislation and several classes of veterinary medicinal products under the Veterinary Medicines Regulations. An understanding of these and associated professional issues is important to pharmacists as medicines should not be considered normal items of commerce, and the final decision on sale or supply is one determined by the professional judgment of the pharmacist

Pharmacists' are empowered to refuse to sell or supply ANY medicines, if the sale or supply is contrary to the pharmacist's clinical judgment.

There will be different situations requiring varying levels of explanation as to why a sale or supply was refused. This will depend upon whether or not it is the patient who is asking and if not whether the person asking has clinical expertise and a legitimate interest.

FURTHER RESOURCES

An A–Z list of medicines for human use and their legal classification is available to members on the Royal Pharmaceutical Society website (**www.rpharms.com**).

GSL medicines

General sales list (GSL) medicines are those that can be sold in registered pharmacies but also in other retail outlets that can 'close so as to exclude the public'. They are classified as GSL mostly because of an EU or UK marketing authorisation (product licence), if they hold a traditional herbal registration or if they have a certificate of registration as a GSL homeopathic product.

The term (PO) medicine is sometimes used by manufacturers as a term that describes a product that is licensed as a GSL medicine but for which the manufacturer wishes to restrict sales or supplies through pharmacies only (e.g. 30-sachet packs of Fybogel).

Within a pharmacy, GSL medicines can only be sold when a pharmacist has assumed the role of responsible pharmacist; however, the pharmacist may be physically absent for a limited period of time while remaining responsible, thus permitting sales of GSL medicines during this absence (see Appendix 10).

Pharmacy (P) medicines

A pharmacy medicine is a medicinal product that can be sold from a registered pharmacy premises by a pharmacist or a person acting under the supervision of a pharmacist.

Together with GSL medicines, P medicines are collectively known as over-the-counter (OTC) or non-prescription medicines. The sale of some of these medicines is associated with additional legal and professional considerations; the most common issues are explained in section 3.2.

Prescription–only medicines (POM)

A prescription-only medicine (POM) is a medicine that is generally subject to the restriction of requiring a prescription written by an appropriate practitioner (doctor, dentist, supplementary prescriber, nurse independent prescriber, pharmacist independent prescriber, EEA and Swiss doctors and dentists (but not for all controlled drugs), community practitioner nurses (for a limited selection of POMs), optometrist independent prescribers (not for controlled drugs, or parenteral medicines) before it can be sold or supplied. There are exemptions to requiring a prescription in some circumstances (see section 3.3.9). Further details about the legal and professional issues associated with POMs are discussed in section 3.3.

Some medicines can be classified under more than one category and this can depend upon formulation, strength, quantity, indication or marketing authorisation.

3.2 Professional and legal issues: pharmacy medicines

3.2.1 PSEUDOEPHEDRINE AND EPHEDRINE

3.2.2 OTC ORAL EMERGENCY CONTRACEPTION

3.2.3 PARACETAMOL AND ASPIRIN

3.2.4 CODEINE AND DIHYDROCODEINE

3.2.5 COUGH AND COLD MEDICINES FOR CHILDREN

3.2.6 RECLASSIFIED MEDICINES

3.2.1 PSEUDOEPHEDRINE AND EPHEDRINE

Pseudoephedrine and ephedrine are widely used decongestant pharmacy medicines. However, due to their potential for misuse in the illicit production of methylamphetamine (crystal meth) – a class A controlled drug – there are legal restrictions on the quantities that can be sold or supplied without prescription. A class A drug is associated with the most severe penalties for possession and dealing.

- It is unlawful to supply a product or combination of products that contain more than 720mg of pseudoephedrine OR 180mg of ephedrine at any one time, without a prescription

- It is unlawful to sell or supply any pseudoephedrine product at the same time as an ephedrine product without a prescription

Sales or supplies of pseudoephedrine or ephedrine should either be made personally by the pharmacist or by pharmacy staff who have been trained and are competent to deal with pseudoephedrine and ephedrine issues, and who know when it is necessary to refer to the pharmacist.

Even when a request is made for a lawful quantity, the sale or supply can be refused where there are reasonable grounds for suspecting misuse. A person purchasing pseudoephedrine and ephedrine for illicit purposes may not be a 'user' of methylamphetamine and, therefore, may not conform to stereotypes. They may be male, female and of any age or background.

Suspicions can be reported to your local GPhC inspector, local controlled drugs liaison police officer or accountable officer.

SIGNS OF POSSIBLE MISUSE

The following signs in combination can be useful for identifying when a request is more likely to be suspicious.

- **NERVOUS OR GUILTY BEHAVIOUR –** avoiding eye contact, appearing to be uncomfortable answering questions, unusually timid

- **LACK OF SYMPTOMS –** not suffering from cough, cold or flu symptoms, or unable to describe these in the patient if buying for someone else

- **REHEARSED ANSWERS –** gives answers that appear to be rehearsed or scripted

- **IMPATIENT OR AGGRESSIVE –** in a rush or hurrying to complete the transaction

- **OPPORTUNISTIC –** waiting for busy periods in the shop or until less experienced staff are available

- **SPECIFIC PRODUCTS –** wants certain brands that contain only pseudoephedrine or ephedrine

- **PARAPHERNALIA –** wishes also to purchase other items which can be used to manufacture methylamphetamine (e.g. lithium batteries, chemicals such as acetone)

- **QUANTITIES –** requests large quantities

- **FREQUENCY –** makes frequent requests

FURTHER READING

RPS Support. *Pseudoephedrine and ephedrine – quick reference guide.* 2010. (**www.rpharms.com**)

Levonorgestrel 1500 microgram oral emergency hormonal contraception (EHC) is licensed as a pharmacy medicine for women aged 16 years or over. Although the medicine is an OTC product, the pharmacist should be involved in assessing suitability and approving sales.

Advance supply of levonorgestrel-containing oral EHC

Pharmacists can provide an advance supply of levonorgestrel oral EHC (i.e. prior to unprotected sexual intercourse or in case of failure of a contraceptive method) to a patient requesting it at a pharmacy. The patient should be assessed to ensure that they are competent, they intend to use the medicine appropriately and it is clinically appropriate.

Religious or moral beliefs

See Appendix 8 for provisional GPhC guidance on the provision of pharmacy services affected by religious or moral beliefs.

Vulnerable adults and children

Be aware that, in some circumstances, requests for EHC could be linked to abuse (non-consensual intercourse) of children or vulnerable adults. The Department of Health has published a document called "Responding to domestic abuse: A handbook for health professionals", which provides practical advice on dealing with domestic abuse, keeping records, confidentiality and sharing information.

The Department for Education has published a guidance document called "Working together to safeguard children", which includes sections for health professionals and on referral.

Other mechanisms for supply

There are various mechanisms for the supply of EHC and it may be appropriate to refer to other service providers rather than make a sale, in some circumstances (e.g. where a sale would be outside of the terms of the marketing authorisation). Other providers include family planning clinics, general practice clinics and providers of PGDs for EHC and genitourinary medicine (GUM) clinics.

FURTHER READING

RPS Support. *Oral emergency contraception – quick reference guide.* 2011. (**www.rpharms.com**)

Online resources are available from the Faculty of Sexual & Reproductive Healthcare website (**www.ffprhc.org.uk**)

Department for Education. *Working together to safeguard children.* March 2010. (Available at **www.education.gov.uk**) (accessed 24 May 2011)

Online resources are available from the National Society for the Prevention of Cruelty to Children website (**www.nspcc.org.uk**). The society also has a helpline (tel: 0800 800 500)

Department of Health. *Responding to domestic abuse: A handbook for health professionals.* December 2005. Available at (**www.dh.gov.uk**) (accessed on 24 May 2011)

Centre for Pharmacy Postgraduate Education. *Emergency contraception.* 2005. (**www.cppe.ac.uk**) (accessed 24 May 2011)

3.2.3 PARACETAMOL AND ASPIRIN

Paracetamol and aspirin are medicinal products that are available in a range of formulations, strengths and packaged quantities. They have marketing authorisations as POM, P and GSL medicines – depending upon pack size and formulation. Legal restrictions on the total quantities of certain formulations of these medicines that can be sold without prescription have been deemed necessary. Table 1 illustrates the quantities of paracetamol and aspirin that can be sold legally.

TABLE 1: PARACETAMOL AND ASPIRIN – OTC LEGAL RESTRICTIONS

	LEGAL RESTRICTION	ADDITIONAL NOTE
PARACETAMOL	Not more than 100 non-effervescent* tablets or capsules can be sold to a person at any one time. Since most OTC pack sizes are for 16 or 32 dose units, this means that, in practice, less than 100 non-effervescent tablets or capsules can be sold	There are no legal limits on the quantity of over-the-counter effervescent* tablets, powders, granules or liquids that can be sold to a person at any one time. Use professional judgment to decide the appropriate quantity to supply and what limits to impose
ASPIRIN	Not more than 100 non-effervescent* tablets or capsules can be sold to a person at any one time. Since most OTC pack sizes are for 16 or 32 dose units, this means that, in practice, less than 100 non-effervescent tablets or capsules can be sold	There are no legal limits on the quantities of over-the-counter effervescent* tablets or powders that can be sold to a person at any one time. Use professional judgment to decide the appropriate quantity to supply and what limits to impose

* NB The definition of effervescent for the purposes of the restrictions above is provided by medicines legislation. Soluble or dispersible formulations as defined by the British Pharmacopoeia may not meet the definition of effervescent in medicines legislation. Where in doubt, quantities of soluble or dispersible formulations sold should be restricted as non-effervescent preparations.

3.2.4 CODEINE AND DIHYDROCODEINE

In September 2009, the Medicines and Healthcare products Regulatory Agency (MHRA) announced that there would be tighter controls and new warnings on packaging of OTC solid dose medicines (e.g. tablet and capsules) containing codeine or dihydrocodeine. These were introduced to minimise the risk of overuse and addiction of these medicines.

The necessary changes to marketing authorisations (product licences) for pre-existing OTC codeine and dihydrocodeine medicines were completed by 31 December 2009. From the date that the marketing authorisation was changed, all new batches would have been manufactured and labelled with the new warnings and subject to the tighter controls.

The changes include:

- **INDICATIONS** – indications for solid dose OTC codeine and dihydrocodeine products are now restricted to the short-term treatment of acute, moderate pain that is not relieved by paracetamol, ibuprofen or aspirin alone. All other previous indications, including cold, flu, cough, sore throats and minor pain have been removed

- **PACK SIZES** – any pack containing more than 32 dose units now requires a marketing authorisation as a POM. This includes effervescent formulations

- **PILS AND LABELS** – the warning "Can cause addiction. For three days use only" must now be positioned in a prominent clear position on the front of the pack. In addition, both the PIL and packaging need to state the indication and that the medicine can cause addiction or overuse headache if used continuously for more than three days. The PIL must also contain information about the warning signs of addiction

The RPS supports the purpose of these tighter controls and recommend that only one pack of OTC medication containing codeine or dihydrocodeine should be sold as sale of more than one pack would undermine the reduction in pack size and POM restriction on packs containing more than 32 dose units.

Updated packaging and product information will have been available since June 2010.

Pre-existing packs marked as 'P' products, which are intended by the manufacturers to be used for dispensing purposes only (e.g. packs of 100 effervescent paracetamol and codeine), should not be sold as OTC medicines.

3.2.5 COUGH AND COLD MEDICINES FOR CHILDREN

In 2009 the Commission on Human Medicines reviewed the evidence for using cough and cold medicines in children and found that there were limited studies to support this use. These medicines had been introduced in the past when requirements to demonstrate safety and efficacy were less demanding than they were in 2009.

As a result, the MHRA issued important advice affecting the use of cough and cold medicines in children aged below 12, which resulted in significant changes to the marketing authorisations for these medicines.

Many cough and cold medicines are no longer used in children under six years of age as there is no evidence that they are effective and, in some cases, the ingredients are linked to side effects including allergies, sleep disturbances and hallucinations.

Medicines containing the following ingredients have been deemed unsuitable for children:

- **ANTITUSSIVES** – dextromethorphan, pholcodine
- **EXPECTORANTS** – guaifenesin, ipecacuanha
- **NASAL DECONGESTANTS** – ephedrine, oxymetazoline, phenylephrine, pseudoephedrine, xylometazoline
- **ANTIHISTAMINES** – brompheniramine, chlorphenamine, diphenhydramine, doxylamine, promethazine, triprolidine

Where these medicines still hold marketing authorisations they are now indicated for use as second line to best practice (see below) and should not be used for more than five days. Warning labels on the packaging and labelling for these medicines have been strengthened to reflect the 2009 advice.

There is also an ongoing change to ensure that all liquid cough and cold medicines are supplied in a child-resistant container.

Useful lists (non-exhaustive) of the medicinal products that can be sold or supplied for use by children under six years of age, and for children aged between six and 12 years, are available on the RPS website (**www.rpharms.com**).

Best practice for treating children with a cough and/or a cold

Most colds will resolve within five to seven days. However, the following treatment or advice can be given as first-line remedies if the symptoms are causing discomfort or distress. All medicines must also be given in accordance with licensed indications:

- **FOR ALL SYMPTOMS** – non-pharmacological interventions such as advising that the child drinks plenty of fluids
- **FOR FEVER AND PAIN** – treat with paracetamol or ibuprofen. National Institute for Health and Clinical Excellence (NICE) guidelines (**www.nice.org.uk**) do not currently recommend using paracetamol and ibuprofen at the same time in children under five years. Currently, the second of these medicines should only be considered if the child does not respond to the first
- **FOR NASAL CONGESTION** – treat with saline nasal drops, vapour rubs or decongestants, or steam inhalation

- **FOR A COUGH** – warm, clear fluids or warm lemon and honey drinks can be advised if the child is aged over one year. Also, simple cough mixtures such as glycerol or simple linctus can be recommended

If symptoms persist or you suspect that it may be a more serious condition, refer the patient to their GP.

Sale of medicines containing the listed ingredients for indications other than cough and cold

Medicines containing those ingredients listed above can continue to be sold for use in children for licensed indications other than cough and cold. For example, Piriton (chlorpheniramine) is not licensed for treating a cough or cold so should not be sold for this purpose. However, it can be sold for its licensed uses.

Codeine linctus for dry, unproductive coughs in children and young people

The MHRA issued new advice in October 2010 that OTC liquid preparations containing codeine should not be used in children or young people under 18 years because the risks outweigh the benefits. This affects all codeine linctus BP products that are currently licensed for use in those under 18 years (including Pulmo Bailly, Galcodine linctus and Galcodine paediatric linctus). Codeine products containing new packaging leaflets became available from April 2011 and the introduction of child resistant containers is anticipated by June 2012.

FURTHER READING

Department of Health. *Birth to Five* (2009 edition). October 2009. (**www.dh.gov.uk**) (accessed 24 May 2011)

Online resources are available on the NHS Choices website (**www.nhs.uk**)

RPS Support. *Children's cough and cold – quick reference guide.* 2010. Available at the Royal Pharmaceutical Society (**www.rpharms.com**)

Online resources are available on the MHRA website (**www.mhra.gov.uk**)

National Institute for Health and Clinical Excellence. *Feverish illness in children.* May 2007. **www.nice.org.uk** (accessed on 24 May 2011)

3.2.6 RECLASSIFIED MEDICINES

Increasingly, more medicines are being reclassified from POM to P, providing pharmacists with a larger repertoire of medicines to select from to treat patients. It is appropriate that pharmacists involved in the sale of reclassified medicines are appropriately trained on relevant clinical and best practice aspects of the medicines and that pharmacy support staff are trained and/or work under protocols (as appropriate) when they supply these medicines. This is particularly relevant to newly reclassified POM to P medicines but also applies to all reclassifications and P medicines generally.

FURTHER RESOURCES

Information on legal status, reclassification, and lists of reclassified medicines are available on the MHRA website (**www.mhra.gov.uk**; search for "Legal status of medicines")

Guidance for the following reclassified medicines is available from the RPS website (**www.rpharms.com**; search for "Reclassifications"):

Amorolfine nail lacquer
Azithromycin
Chloramphenicol eye drops
Omeprazole
Orlistat
Sumatriptan
Tamsulosin
Tranexamic acid

3.3 Professional and legal issues: prescription-only medicines

3.3.1   GENERAL PRESCRIPTION REQUIREMENTS

3.3.2   FAXED PRESCRIPTIONS

3.3.3   DENTAL PRESCRIPTIONS

3.3.4   FORGED PRESCRIPTIONS

3.3.5   PRESCRIPTIONS FROM THE EEA OR SWITZERLAND

3.3.6   LABELLING OF DISPENSED MEDICINAL PRODUCTS

3.3.7   ADMINISTRATION

3.3.8   PATIENT SPECIFIC DIRECTIONS AND ADMINISTRATION, SALE OR SUPPLY IN HOSPITALS AND OTHER SETTINGS

3.3.9   EXEMPTIONS: SALE AND SUPPLY WITHOUT A PRESCRIPTION

3.3.10 SELF-PRESCRIBED PRESCRIPTIONS AND PRESCRIPTIONS FOR CLOSE FRIENDS AND FAMILY

3.3.11 SUPPLYING ISOTRETINOIN AND PREGNANCY PREVENTION

3.3.12 SUMMARY OF PRESCRIBER TYPES AND PRESCRIBING RESTRICTIONS

3.3.1 GENERAL PRESCRIPTION REQUIREMENTS

The sale, supply and administration of prescription-only medicines (POMs) are restricted by legislation. The main route by which a pharmacist is able to sell or supply a POM is under the authority of a prescription from an appropriate practitioner (doctor, dentist, supplementary prescriber, nurse independent prescriber, pharmacist independent prescriber, EEA and Swiss doctors and dentists (but not for all CDs), community practitioner nurses (for a limited selection of POMs), optometrist independent prescribers (not for CDs, or parenteral medicines), or via an exemption (see section 3.3.9).

NB: The additional prescription requirements for controlled drugs are discussed in section 3.7.7.

Several pieces of information must be present for a prescription to be legal. These are specified in Diagram 3.

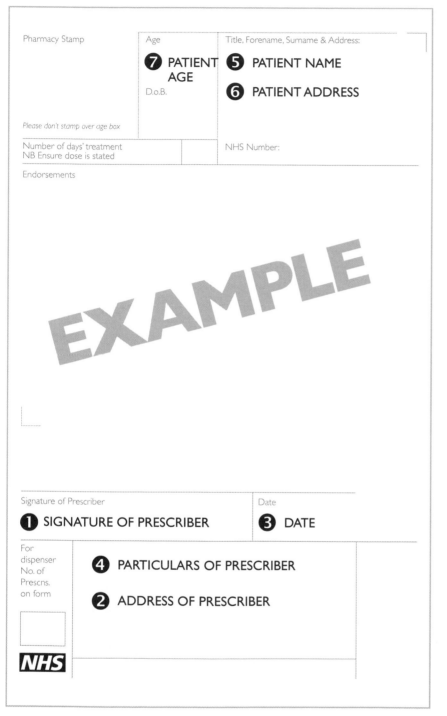

Pharmacy Stamp

Age
7 PATIENT AGE
D.o.B.

Title, Forename, Surname & Address:
5 PATIENT NAME
6 PATIENT ADDRESS

Please don't stamp over age box

Number of days' treatment
NB Ensure dose is stated

NHS Number:

Endorsements

EXAMPLE

Signature of Prescriber
1 SIGNATURE OF PRESCRIBER

Date
3 DATE

For dispenser No. of Prescns. on form

4 PARTICULARS OF PRESCRIBER

2 ADDRESS OF PRESCRIBER

NHS

DIAGRAM 3: PRESCRIPTION REQUIREMENTS

NB: Indelible – Prescriptions need to be written in indelible ink; they may be computer generated or typed

NB: Private prescriptions – The diagram above bears the image of an NHS prescription; however, the same requirements apply to private prescriptions

1 SIGNATURE – prescriptions need to be signed in indelible ink by an appropriate practitioner (see 3.3.1) in his or her own name. An 'advanced electronic signature' can be used to authorise an electronic prescription; this is a signature that is linked uniquely to the signatory, capable of identifying the signatory and created using means over which the signatory can maintain sole control. The Royal Pharmaceutical Society is unable to confirm whether or not individual systems are able to issue advanced electronic signatures. Suitable assurances should be obtained from the system manufacturer and business indemnity providers

2 ADDRESS – prescriptions must include the address of the appropriate practitioner (see 3.3.1)

3 DATE – prescriptions need to include the date on which they were signed; a prescription is valid for up to six months from the *appropriate* date (for prescriptions for schedules 2, 3 or 4 controlled drugs, see section 3.7.7). The appropriate date is the later of either the date on which the prescription was signed or a date indicated by the appropriate practitioner (see 3.3.1) as the date before which it should not be dispensed

4 PARTICULARS – prescriptions require particulars that indicate the type of appropriate practitioner (see 3.3.1)

5 NAME OF THE PATIENT

6 ADDRESS OF THE PATIENT (not required for prescriptions written by EEA or Swiss prescribers)

7 AGE OF THE PATIENT if under 12 years old (not required for prescriptions written by EEA or Swiss prescribers)

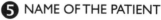

Repeatable prescriptions

Repeatable prescriptions are prescriptions against which medicines can be dispensed more than once. NHS prescriptions and prescriptions for schedule 2 or 3 controlled drugs are not repeatable.

Private prescriptions can be repeated as indicated by the prescriber (e.g. repeat × 3) but if the number of repeats is not stated then they can only be repeated once. The only exception to this is a prescription for an oral contraceptive, which can be dispensed six times (i.e. repeated five times) within six months of the appropriate date (see above). For other repeatable prescriptions, the first dispensing must be made within six months of the appropriate date, following which there is no legal time limit for the remaining repeats. However, pharmacists should use professional judgment, taking into consideration clinical factors, to determine whether further repeat dispensing is appropriate.

NB: Repeatable prescriptions are a different concept from repeat prescribing for regular items made under the NHS repeat dispensing scheme (in England and Wales), and also different to instalment prescribing for controlled drugs (see section 3.7.7) or where the counterpart section of prescriptions used by patients to order 'repeats' of their prescription from the prescriber.

Prisons provide NHS healthcare for their patients and so any prescriptions written for prisoners cannot be repeated unless they fall under an NHS repeat dispensing scheme.

Record keeping

Private prescriptions for a POM must be retained for two years from the date of the last sale or supply. Records must be made in the POM register and must include:

- **SUPPLY DATE** – the date on which the medicine was sold or supplied

- **PRESCRIPTION DATE** – the date on the prescription

- **MEDICINE DETAILS** – the name, quantity, formulation and strength of medicine supplied (where not apparent from the name)

- **PRESCRIBER DETAILS** – the name and address of the practitioner

- **PATIENT DETAILS** – the name and address of the patient

Prescriptions for oral contraceptives are exempt from record keeping; as are prescriptions for schedule 2 controlled drugs where a separate controlled register record has been made (see section 3.7.11).

Incomplete prescriptions

Details of the medicinal product (such as name, strength, form, quantity and dose) are not legal requirements for prescriptions for POMs. Clearly, however, they are important for identifying which medicine to supply, how much to supply and at what dose. It is also important from a prescription pricing and remuneration perspective.

Information on appropriate steps to take when an incomplete prescription is received is available in the "Guidance on prescribing" section at the start of the British National Formulary (**www.bnf.org**).

PRESCRIPTIONS FOR DISCHARGED PRISONERS – ENGLAND

FP10 prescriptions are not allowed for patients while they are in prison. However, those who are about to be discharged from prison without the usual methods for ensuring continuity of supply of their medicines (e.g. those released unexpectedly from court, those who fail to obtain a take-out supply of their medicines or those who fail to obtain a same or next day prescribing appointment with a drug treatment agency) can be given an FP10 or FP10[MDA] prescription to take to their community pharmacy. These FP10 forms have the name and address of the prison printed on them and the patient is exempt from payment by virtue of having HMP in the address.

For more information, the Department of Health has produced guidance entitled "Provision of FP10 and FP10[MDA] prescription forms by HM Prison Service for released prisoners" (available at **www.dh.gov.uk**).

3.3.2 FAXED PRESCRIPTIONS

A 'fax' of a prescription does not fall within the definition of a legally valid prescription within human medicines legislation because it is not written in indelible ink and has not been signed by an appropriate practitioner. Supplying medicines against a 'fax' is associated with considerable risks;

1. Uncertainty that the supply has been made in accordance with a legally valid prescription

2. Risks of poor reproduction

3. Risks of non-receipt of the original prescription and therefore inability to demonstrate that a supply had been made in accordance with a prescription

4. Risks that the original prescription is subsequently amended by the prescriber in which case the supply would not have been made in accordance with the prescription

5. Risks the 'fax' is sent to multiple pharmacies and duplicate supplies are made

6. Risks that the prescription is not genuine

7. Risks that the system of sending and receiving of the 'fax' is not secure

Alternative mechanisms for the supply of medicines in an emergency exist for pharmacists working in registered pharmacies and can achieve a similar outcome in many scenarios with a better risk profile. Where this option can be used, it should be used.

Electronic prescriptions are also recognised in medicines legislation and where a system is being developed should be considered as an option.

Pharmacists considering supplying medicines against a fax should make an informed decision and take steps to safeguard patient safety, and where possible mitigate the risks identified above.

The supply of schedule 2 and 3 controlled drugs without possession of a lawful prescription could be prosecuted as a criminal offence.

FURTHER RESOURCES

Further information on additional safeguards used in sectors such as 'secure environments' and secondary care maybe available from specialist groups (see section 6) or from the specialist virtual networks on the RPS website (**www.rpharms.com**)

The Pharmaceutical Services Negotiations Committee also has additional information available online within their 'Internet Pharmacy FAQ' document (**www.psnc.org.uk**)

3.3.3 DENTAL PRESCRIPTIONS

Dentists can write prescriptions legally for any POM. However, they should restrict their prescribing to areas in which they are competent and generally only prescribe medicines that have uses in dentistry.

When prescribing on an NHS dental prescription, dentists are restricted to the medicines listed in the Dental

Prescribers' Formulary (Part 8a of the Drug Tariff for Scotland or Part XVIIa of the Drug Tariff for England and Wales). The dental formulary is also reproduced within the British National Formulary.

3.3.4 FORGED PRESCRIPTIONS

Although it can be difficult to detect a forged prescription, every pharmacist should be alert to the possibility that any prescription could be a forgery.

The following checklist may be useful to help detect fraudulent prescriptions and prompt further investigation:

- Is a large or excessive quantity prescribed and is this appropriate for the medicine and condition being treated?
- Is the prescriber known?
- Is the patient known?
- Has the title 'Dr' been inserted before the signature?
- Is the behaviour of the patient indicative? (e.g. nervous, agitated, aggressive, etc)
- Is the medicine known to be commonly misused?

Further investigation may be necessary. The following are appropriate actions to take:

1. Scrutinise the signature carefully – possibly checking against a known genuine prescription from the same prescriber

2. Confirm details with the prescriber (e.g. whether or not a prescription has been issued, the original intention of the prescriber and whether or not there has been an alteration)

3. Use contact details for the prescriber that are obtained from a source other than the suspicious prescription (e.g. Directory Enquiries)

Reporting concerns

Depending upon the nature of the fraudulent prescription, use your professional judgment to assess whether or not it is a matter that requires referral to the police, NHS Counter Fraud Services (for NHS prescriptions only) or whether the matter can be resolved by discussions with the patient and prescriber.

FURTHER READING

Further information on NHS Counter Fraud Services is available at (**www.nhsbsa.nhs.uk/CounterFraud.aspx**) (accessed 27 May 2011)

Further information on NHS Scotland Counter Fraud Services is available at (**www.cfs.scot.nhs.uk**)

3.3.5 PRESCRIPTIONS FROM THE EEA OR SWITZERLAND

Since November 2008, valid prescriptions issued by a doctor or dentist registered in an EEA country (for a list of EEA countries see below) or Switzerland have been legally recognised in the UK. Emergency supplies for patients of doctors and dentists registered in an EEA country or Switzerland was also enabled at the same time.

LIST OF EEA COUNTRIES

Austria, Belgium, Bulgaria, Cyprus, Czech Republic, Denmark, Estonia, Finland, France, Germany, Greece, Hungary, Iceland, Ireland, Italy, Latvia, Liechtenstein, Lithuania, Luxembourg, Malta, Netherlands, Norway, Poland, Portugal, Romania, Spain, Slovak Republic, Slovenia, Sweden

Prescription requirements

Requirements for prescriptions from the EEA or Switzerland are the same as the usual UK requirements (see section 3.3.1) with the exception that the age and address of the patient are not legal requirements. Even if the prescription requirements have been written in a foreign language the prescription is still legally acceptable. However, the pharmacist must be able to understand the language to dispense the prescribed medicine safely and to be satisfied that the prescription is compliant with legal requirements. An emergency supply or referral to an appropriate UK-registered prescriber could also be options.

Medicines not available on an EEA prescription

Schedule 1, 2 or 3 controlled drugs cannot be dispensed in the UK when prescribed by an EEA or Swiss doctor or dentist. Consider referral to an appropriate UK-registered prescriber if such items are requested.

Checking the registration status of an EEA prescriber

A pan-EEA database of prescribers does not exist and, indeed, not all of the other EEA countries have a register of practitioners or online registers in English. Therefore, it may not always be possible to check the registration of an EEA prescriber. However, up-to-date contact details for EEA competent authorities can be found for doctors on the General Medical Council website (**www.gmc-uk.org**; search for "EEA evidence of qualifications") and for dentists on the General Dental Council website (**www.gdc-uk.org**; search for "List of EEA competent authorities").

Inability to confirm registration status

If it is not possible to confirm the registration status of the EEA prescriber after taking all reasonable steps to do so, then it may still be possible to make a safe and legal supply in the interests of patient care. It would be beneficial to keep a record of the details of any interventions and steps taken. This would require checking (and being satisfied) that prescription requirements are fulfilled, questioning the patient and careful use of professional judgment. A 'due diligence' defence exists for EEA prescriptions. However, only a court could decide, ultimately on a case-by-case basis, whether due diligence has been exercised.

Emergency supply

Emergency supplies at the request of a patient, or at the request of the EEA or Swiss prescriber, are legally possible. The usual emergency supply process (see section 3.3.9.2) should be used and, where the request originates from an EEA prescriber, then a prescription needs to be received within 72 hours. Remember that schedule 1, 2 and 3 (including phenobarbital) cannot be supplied to a patient of an EEA or Swiss prescriber as an emergency supply.

Referral

It is important to bear in mind that the legislation outlined above is enabling – it is not obligatory to dispense an EEA prescription if presented with one. If a pharmacist is not satisfied that a prescription is clinically appropriate, or legally valid, and an emergency supply is not appropriate, then a valid alternative remains to refer the patient to a doctor or dentist based in the UK.

3.3.6 LABELLING OF DISPENSED MEDICINAL PRODUCTS

When a medicinal product is dispensed there is a legal requirement for the following to appear on the dispensing label:

- Name of the patient
- Name and address of the supplying pharmacy
- Date of dispensing
- Name of the medicine
- Directions for use
- Precautions relating to the use of the medicine
- The words "Keep out of the reach of children"
- Where applicable, the words "For external use only"

NB: In secure environments it is strongly recommended that the prisoner number is also included on the label as a definitive patient identifier.

Additional information can be added to the dispensing label if the pharmacist considers it to be necessary.

OUTER CONTAINER Whilst it is lawful to label the outer container, we advise that the labelling recommendations of the National Patient Safety Agency are followed. These guidelines raise the issue that the outer container may be discarded and, therefore, the labelling information could be lost, so the actual container (e.g. inhaler or tube of cream) should be labelled rather than the outer container

OPTIMISATION OF LABELLING If it is the professional opinion of the pharmacist that either the 'directions for use' or 'name of the medicine' or 'precautions relating to the use of the medicine' are not appropriate, then these may be substituted with more suitable particulars of a similar kind. At the time of writing, this can only take place having attempted to consult with the prescriber. It is expected that the requirement to check with the prescriber in advance will not be required once the consolidation and review of the Medicines Act and the Human Medicines Regulations are in force. This will not enable generic substitution and permits pharmacists to make changes to the dispensing label as outlined above. It would be good practice to make a record of the intervention. The option to contact the prescriber for clarification, prior to making a supply remains available.

Labelling requirements for pre-packed or assembled medicines

Pharmacists are able to break down bulk containers into smaller quantities more appropriate for dispensing against prescriptions in anticipation of these prescriptions. These must be labelled with the:

- Name of the medicine
- Quantity of the medicine in the container (i.e. the ingredients)

3.3.7 ADMINISTRATION

Medicines legislation prevents a person administering a parenteral POM to another person unless they are acting in accordance with the directions of an appropriate practitioner. However there are exemptions to this restriction.

- Quantitative particulars of the medicines (i.e. the ingredients)
- Handling and storage requirements where appropriate
- Expiry date
- Batch reference number (e.g. LOT number or BN number)

Upon dispensing, these pre-packed medicines need to be labelled with the usual labelling requirements.

NB: Packing and supplying to a separate legal entity (e.g. for an NHS trust to supply a different NHS trust or an out-of-hours medical practice) is not permitted without an assembly licence from the MHRA (which require additional conditions). The MHRA can be contacted for further details (**www.mhra.gov.uk**).

Manufacturer labelling requirements

Apart from the requirements that need to appear on a dispensing label, legislation also underpins the labelling requirements that appear on a container of a medicinal product for manufacturers. These details are outside of the scope of this guide. However, further information can be obtained from the document "Best practice guidance on labelling and packaging of medicines", which can be found on the MHRA website (**www.mhra.gov.uk**).

Medicines legislation allows the administration of listed parenteral medicines to human beings in an emergency for the purpose of saving life. This allows the following parenteral medicines to be administered in an emergency by any person (adrenaline, atropine sulphate, chlorphenamine, dicobalt edetate, glucagon, glucose, hydrocortisone, naloxone, pralidoxine, promethazine, snake venom antiserum, sodium nitrate and sodium thiosulphate).

This is an indicative list only and full details will be available within the Human Medicines Regulations 2012.

Further exemptions apply to the administration of smallpox vaccine or administration linked to medical exposure (including radioactive medicines), and to specific classes

of persons (such as midwives and paramedics) for specified parenteral POMs under certain conditions.

Medicines legislation does not restrict who can administer a non-parenteral POMs (i.e. oral, inhaled, topical or rectal dosage forms, etc). However, in most healthcare settings, the person administering the medicine should only do so with the authority of a prescription, patient specific direction or patient group direction and should be appropriately trained.

3.3.8 PATIENT SPECIFIC DIRECTIONS AND ADMINISTRATION, SALE AND SUPPLY IN HOSPITALS AND OTHER SETTINGS

Medicines legislation provides a range of exemptions to the restrictions on the sale, supply and administration of medicines.

A number of these exemptions are collectively described as patient specific directions (PSDs).

Legislation does not specifically define a PSD. However, it is generally accepted to mean a written instruction from a doctor, dentist or other independent prescriber for a medicine to be supplied or administered to a named patient after the prescriber has assessed that patient on an individual basis.

Some organisations may limit who is authorised to supply and/or administer medicines under a PSD within their local medicines policies and governance arrangements. Any trained and competent health professional would be suitable. PSDs relate to a specific named patient but do not need to comply with the requirements specified for a prescription.

In a hospital ward, written PSDs are encountered on inpatient charts as directions to administer. While the law does not stipulate what should be included in a PSD, sufficient information must be available for the person administering the specified medicine to do so safely. In addition a PSD, if sufficiently clear, may also be a direction to make a sale or supply.

Typically the directions within an inpatient chart are transcribed onto an order form for the pharmacy to prepare discharge ('take home') medicines. This may take the form of an electronic or hard copy discharge letter. The pharmacist in this instance is not prescribing, and the supply is made under the authority of the original written direction to supply. Transcription should be carried out or counter-checked by a pharmacist.

For the purpose of administration (rather than supply) it is also possible for the directions of an appropriate practitioner to be verbal or telephoned. This is because medicines legislation does not specify that the authorisation to administer a medicine needs to be in writing. Nevertheless, a written authorisation should be used wherever possible and any applicable standards that require the authorisation to be in writing should be adhered to. For example, in England, the Care Quality Commission essential standards for quality and safety, and the standards of any relevant healthcare professionals involved in administration (e.g. nurses) will be applicable.

Some hospitals have formulated policies to permit, in an emergency, the administration of medicines following a telephoned or verbal request from an appropriate practitioner – usually involving two nurses checking one another.

Some hospitals have also formulated policies for the supply and/or administration of POMs (and P or GSL medicines) to ensure that medicines are handled safely, securely and appropriately. Such policies should be carefully considered and agreed by medical, nursing and pharmacy staff to ensure that patients are not put at risk. The policy should be cross-referenced against standards set by any applicable body, including regulatory and professional bodies of relevant healthcare professionals involved in the process. If in doubt, the Department of Health should be consulted for hospitals in England (along with the hospital's legal advisors). Hospitals in Scotland should contact the Scottish Executive, while hospitals in Wales should contact the Department of Health and Social Services.

British Medical Association. *Patient group directions and patient specific directions in general practice.* August 2010. (**www.bma.org.uk**)

Dale A. *Patient specific directions: Brief Q and A on their use.* March 2009. (**www.nelm.nhs.uk**)

Online resources are available on the NHS Education for Scotland website (**www.nes.scot.nhs.uk**)

Department of Health. *Medicine matters: A guide to mechanisms for the prescribing, supply and administration of medicines.* March 2005. (**www.dh.gov.uk**)

Online resources are available on the Care Quality Commission website (**www.cqc.org.uk**)

Nursing and Midwifery Council. *Standards for medicines management.* 2010.(**www.nmc-uk.org.uk**)

3.3.9 EXEMPTIONS: SALE AND SUPPLY WITHOUT A PRESCRIPTION

3.3.9.1 PATIENT GROUP DIRECTIONS

3.3.9.2 EMERGENCY SUPPLY

3.3.9.3 PANDEMIC EXEMPTIONS

3.3.9.4 OPTOMETRIST SIGNED ORDERS FOR PATIENTS

The preferred way for patients to receive medicines is for an appropriately qualified healthcare professional to prescribe for an individual patient on a one-to-one basis. There are, however, several exemptions that allow POMs to be sold or supplied without a prescription. Pharmacists are likely to be involved in many of these mechanisms and need to be aware of:

■ Patient group directions (PGDs)

■ Patient specific directions (see section 3.3.8)

■ Emergency supplies

■ Pandemic exemptions

■ Optometrist signed orders for patients

3.3.9.1 Patient group directions

A PGD is a written direction that allows the supply and/or administration of a specified medicine or medicines, by named authorised health professionals, to a well-defined group of patients requiring treatment for a specific condition.

It is important that pharmacists involved with PGDs understand the scope and limitations of PGDs as well as the wider context into which they fit to ensure safe, effective services for patients.

The supply and administration of medicines under a PGD should only be reserved for those limited situations where this offers an advantage for patient care, without compromising patient safety. A PGD should only be developed after careful consideration of all the potential methods of supply and/or administration of medicines, including prescribing, by medical or non-medical prescribers.

DEVELOPMENT AND USE OF PGDS DIFFERS IN EACH OF THE HOME NATIONS.

Since the 23 April 2012, pharmacists have been empowered by legislation to supply, offer to supply and administer diamorphine or morphine under PGD for the immediate, necessary treatment of sick or injured persons. Further information about this is available from the NELM PGD website.

Online resources are available at the National Electronic Library for Medicines (NELM) PGD website (England only) (**www.nelm.nhs.uk/ en/Communities/NeLM/PGDs/**)

National Prescribing Centre. *Patient group directions.* December 2009. (**www.npc.nhs.uk**)

NHS Education for Scotland. *Patient group directions.* (**www.nes.scot.nhs.uk/pgds**)

Information on the legal arrangements for NHS and private patient group directions are available on the Medicines and Healthcare products Regulatory Agency website (**www.mhra.gov.uk**)

Centre for Pharmacy Postgraduate Education. *Patient group directions (PGDs) – developing, implementing and using them safely.* 2008. (**www.cppe.ac.uk**)

3.3.9.2 Emergency supply

In an emergency and under certain conditions a pharmacist working in a registered pharmacy can supply POMs to a patient without a prescription if requested by a prescriber or the patient.

In Scotland, a national PGD is in place that allows participating pharmacies and pharmacists to supply medicines for the urgent provision of current repeat medicines, appliances and ACBS (borderline) items. Therefore, pharmacists working in Scotland are only likely to use the standard emergency supply exemptions (outlined below) for patients who are not eligible for treatment under the national PGD. An equivalent national PGD in England and Wales has not been established.

EMERGENCY SUPPLY AT THE REQUEST OF A PRESCRIBER

Doctors, dentists, supplementary prescribers, community practitioner nurse prescribers, nurse independent prescribers, optometrist independent prescribers, pharmacist independent prescribers and EEA or Swiss doctors or dentists can all authorise an emergency supply under certain conditions. The conditions are:

- **APPROPRIATE PRESCRIBER** – the pharmacist is satisfied that the request is from one of the prescribers stated above

- **EMERGENCY** – the pharmacist is satisfied that a prescription cannot be provided immediately due to an emergency

- **PRESCRIPTION WITHIN 72 HOURS** – the prescriber agrees to provide a written prescription within 72 hours

- **DIRECTIONS** – the medicine is supplied in accordance with the direction given by the prescriber

- **NOT FOR CONTROLLED DRUGS, EXCEPT PHENOBARBITAL** – Schedule 1, 2 or 3 controlled drugs cannot be supplied in an emergency with the exception of phenobarbital (also known as phenobarbitone or phenobarbitone sodium) for epilepsy by a UK-registered doctor, dentist, supplementary prescriber and independent pharmacist or nurse prescriber. EEA doctors and dentists cannot request an emergency supply for any schedule 1, 2, or 3 controlled drugs (including phenobarbital for any purpose)

- **RECORD KEPT** – an entry must be made into the POM register on the day of the supply (or, if impractical, on the following day). The entry needs to include:
  - the date the POM was supplied
  - the name (including strength and form where appropriate) and quantity of medicine supplied
  - the name and address of the prescriber requesting the emergency supply
  - the name and address of the patient for whom the POM was required
  - the date on the prescription (this can be added to the entry when the prescription is received by the pharmacy)
  - the date on which the prescription is received (this should be added to the entry when the prescription is received in the pharmacy)

EMERGENCY SUPPLY AT THE REQUEST OF A PATIENT

Emergency supplies are also possible upon the request of a patient from one of the following types of prescriber: doctor, dentist, supplementary prescriber, community practitioner nurse prescriber, nurse independent prescriber, optometrist independent prescriber, pharmacist independent prescriber, and EEA or Swiss doctor or dentist.

The supply can be made in the following circumstances:

- **INTERVIEW** – the pharmacist must interview the patient, preferably face to face (if this is not possible consider using the telephone to contact the patient to gather the relevant information)

- **IMMEDIATE NEED** – the pharmacist must be satisfied that there is an immediate need for the POM and that it is not practical for the patient to obtain a prescription without undue delay

  Legislation does not prevent a pharmacist from making an emergency supply when a doctor's surgery is open. As with any request for an emergency supply, pharmacists must consider the best interests of the patient. Where a pharmacist believes that it would be impracticable in the circumstances for a patient to obtain a prescription without undue delay they may decide that an emergency supply is necessary. Automatically referring patients who are away from home and have forgotten or run out of their medication to the nearest local surgery to register as a temporary resident may not always be the most appropriate course of action

- **PREVIOUS TREATMENT** – the POM requested must previously have been used as a treatment and prescribed by at least one of the types of prescribers listed above

  (NB: The time interval from when the medicine was last prescribed to when it is requested as an emergency supply would need to be considered and you should use your professional judgment to decide whether a supply or referral to a prescriber is appropriate)

- **DOSE** – the pharmacist must be satisfied of knowing the dose that the patient needs to take

- **NOT FOR CONTROLLED DRUGS, EXCEPT PHENOBARBITAL** – phenobarbital can be supplied to patients of UK-registered prescribers for the purpose of treating epilepsy. Medicinal products cannot be supplied if they consist of or contain any other schedule 1, 2 or 3 controlled drugs or the substances listed below: ammonium bromide,

calcium bromide, calcium bromidolactobionate, embutramide, fencamfamin hydrochloride, fluanisone, hexobarbitone, hexobarbitone sodium, hydrobromic acid, meclofenoxate hydrochloride, methohexitone sodium, pemoline, piracetam, potassium bromide, prolintane hydrochloride, sodium bromide, strychnine hydrochloride, tacrine hydrochloride, thiopentone sodium

(NB: Requests made by a patient of an EEA or Swiss doctor/dentist cannot be supplied if they are for medicines that do not have a marketing authorisation valid in the UK – see section 3.3.5)

- **LENGTH OF TREATMENT** – if the emergency supply is for a controlled drug (i.e. phenobarbital or schedule 4 or 5 controlled drug), the maximum quantity that can be supplied is for five days' treatment. For any other POM, no more than 30 days can be supplied except in the following circumstances:

  - if the POM is insulin, an ointment, a cream, or an inhaler for asthma (i.e. the packs cannot be broken), the smallest pack available in the pharmacy should be supplied

  - if the POM is an oral contraceptive, a full treatment cycle should be supplied

  - if the POM is an antibiotic in liquid form for oral administration, the smallest quantity that will provide a full course of treatment should be supplied

  (NB: Pharmacists should also consider whether it is appropriate to supply less than the maximum quantity allowed in legislation. Professional judgment should be used to supply a reasonable quantity that is clinically appropriate and lasts until the patient is able to see a prescriber to obtain a further supply)

- **RECORDS KEPT** – an entry must be made in the POM register on the day of the supply (or, if impractical, on the following day). The entry needs to include:

  - the date the POM was supplied

  - the name (including strength and form where appropriate) and quantity of medicine supplied

  - the name and address of the patient for whom the POM was supplied

  - information on the nature of the emergency, such as why the patient needs the POM and why a prescription cannot be obtained, etc

- **LABELLING** – in addition to standard labelling requirements, the words "Emergency supply" need to be added to the dispensing label

OTHER POINTS TO CONSIDER WHEN FACED WITH REQUESTS FOR AN EMERGENCY SUPPLY

Pharmacists should be mindful of patients abusing emergency supplies (for example, where a patient medication record shows that a patient has requested a medicine as an emergency supply on several occasions).

It is possible to make an emergency supply even during surgery opening hours; trying to obtain a prescription can sometimes cause undue delay in treatment and, potentially, harm to the patient. If patients are away from home and have run out of their medicines, referring them to the nearest surgery to register as a temporary patient may not always be appropriate. An emergency supply can be made provided the conditions above are met.

REFUSAL TO SUPPLY

If a pharmacist decides not to make an emergency supply after gathering and considering the information discussed in this guidance, the patient should be advised on how to obtain a prescription for the medicine or appropriate medical care. This could involve referral to a doctor, NHS walk-in centre or to an Accident and Emergency department.

FURTHER READING

RPS Support. *Emergency supply – quick reference guide.* 2011. (**www.rpharms.com**)

3.3.9.3 Pandemic exemptions

Legislation is in place that relaxes emergency supply requirements in the event of a pandemic or imminent pandemic being declared by the Department of Health. It means that pharmacists would not need to interview the patient who requires a medicine through emergency supply.

Provisions are also in place to allow the supply of medicines against a protocol from designated collection points when a disease is pandemic or imminently pandemic and there is a serious or potentially serious risk to human health. This would require an announcement by the Department of Health in England, the Scottish Government or the Welsh Assembly. These collection points would not need to be registered pharmacy premises and supplies would not need to take place under the supervision of a pharmacist.

Further information is available from the Human Medicines Regulations 2012 which is expected to be in force prior to publication of this edition of MEP.

3.3.9.4 Optometrist or podiatrist signed orders for patients

Optometrists and podiatrists cannot authorise supplies of POMs by writing prescriptions unless they are additionally qualified as independent or supplementary prescribers. However, pharmacists working in registered pharmacies can supply certain POMs directly to patients in accordance with a signed order from any registered optometrist or podiatrist.

If a pharmacist is considering making such a supply, he or she should ensure that the medicine is labelled accordingly as a dispensed medicinal product, a patient information leaflet is supplied to the patient and an appropriate record is made in the POM register. Any additional information or advice that enables the patient to use the medicine safely and effectively should also be provided if it has not already been provided by the optometrist or podiatrist.

FURTHER RESOURCES

The Association of Optometrists (contact details can be found at **www.aop.org.uk**)

MHRA online resources regarding exemptions which apply to optometrists or podiatrists (**www.mhra.gov.uk**)

Pharmacists are occasionally requested to dispense medicines that have been self-prescribed by a prescriber or have been prescribed for close family and friends of the prescriber.

Although a prescription (including one for controlled drugs) in these circumstances may fulfil the usual legal requirements, pharmacists should consider the following before making a supply:

- It is generally considered poor practice to self-prescribe or to prescribe for persons for whom there is a close personal relationship

- The professional judgment of the prescriber may be impaired or influenced by the person they are prescribing for

- It may not be possible for a prescriber to conduct a proper clinical assessment on themselves or on close friends or family

- The regulatory body for doctors (General Medical Council) advises within the "Good Medical Practice" that doctors should not treat themselves and, wherever possible, should avoid providing medical care to anyone with whom they have a close personal relationship

- The regulatory body for nurses (Nursing and Midwifery Council) advises within the document "Standards of proficiency for nurse and midwife prescribers" that nurses and midwives must not prescribe for themselves and, other than in exceptional circumstances, should not prescribe for anyone with whom they have a close personal or emotional relationship

- The existence and content of any local trust, board or hospital policy covering self-prescribing

- The abuse potential of the drug being requested

- Controlled drugs should only be supplied in exceptional circumstances and details documented. Where appropriate, the supply or request may prompt referral to the local controlled drug accountable officer

In an emergency, after exercising professional judgment, a pharmacist may decide that it is appropriate to dispense a medicine that has been self-prescribed or prescribed for persons with whom the prescriber has a close personal relationship.

In the circumstance that refusing to supply is the most appropriate action, be prepared for the person requesting the supply to be disappointed. One strategy would be to clearly and calmly explain that in your professional judgment it would not be appropriate to supply the medicine.

In some circumstances where there is a risk of harm to patients or the public, there may be a duty to raise concerns to the appropriate body (e.g. General Medical Council) (see Appendix 6 for GPhC guidance on raising concerns)

FURTHER READING

Nursing and Midwifery Council. *Standards of proficiency for nurse and midwife prescribers.* April 2006. (**www.nmc-uk.org**)

General Medical Council. *Good medical practice.* November 2006. (**www.gmc-uk.org**)

Isotretinoin is a retinoid: when used orally to treat severe acne it has a high risk of causing severe and serious malformation of a foetus and also increases the risk of spontaneous abortion.

Pharmacists are involved in the dispensing of isotretinoin and in ensuring it is not used by women who might be pregnant or are considering becoming pregnant. A Pregnancy Prevention Programme (PPP) is in place to protect female patients at risk of pregnancy from becoming pregnant whilst using oral isotretinoin, and for at least one month after stopping oral isotretinoin.

The programme is a combination of education for healthcare professionals and patients, therapy management (including pregnancy testing before during and after treatment, contraception requirements) and distribution control.

Therapy should only be initiated by or under the supervision of a consultant dermatologist and under the conditions of the PPP. The prescriber must check that the patient complies with, understands and acknowledges the reasons for pregnancy prevention and agrees to monthly follow-up, contraceptive precautions and pregnancy testing.

Female patients should comply with the PPP conditions unless the prescriber agrees that there are compelling reasons that indicate there is no risk of pregnancy. Reasons may include persons who cannot become pregnant e.g. following a hysterectomy or a female who is not sexually active (and there is certainty that sexual activity will not start during the period of teratogenic risk).

SPECIAL DISTRIBUTION CONTROLS FOR FEMALES AT RISK OF PREGNANCY

1. **PRESCRIPTION VALIDITY** Under the PPP, prescriptions are valid only for seven days and ideally should be dispensed on the date the prescription is written. Prescriptions which are presented after seven days should be considered expired and the patient should be referred back to the prescriber for a new prescription. Pregnancy status may need to be reconfirmed by a further negative pregnancy test

2. **QUANTITY** Check that the quantity is for a maximum of 30 days' supply. A quantity for more than 30 days can only be dispensed if the patient is confirmed by the prescriber as not being under the Pregnancy Prevention Programme

In accordance with MHRA approved guidance, pharmacists should not accept repeat prescriptions, free sample distribution, or faxed prescriptions for oral isotretinoin. A telephone request should only be accepted if this is an emergency supply at the request of a PPP specialist prescriber together with confirmation that pregnancy status has been established as negative within the preceding seven days.

FURTHER RESOURCES

Full details of isotretinoin pregnancy prevention programmes are available on the 'Summary of Product Characteristics' for the oral isotretinoin preparation Available at (**www.medicines.org.uk**)

British National Formulary (**www.bnf.org**)

MHRA online isotretinoin and pregnancy prevention resources for doctors, pharmacists and patients (**www.mhra.gov.uk**)

RPS Support. *Dispensing oral isotretinoin and pregnancy prevention.* 2012. (**www.rpharms.com**)

UNDERPINNING KNOWLEDGE

TABLE 2: THE DIFFERENT TYPES OF PRESCRIBER AND RESTRICTIONS
ON WHAT CAN BE PRESCRIBED

(All columns subject to considerations in other columns)

TYPE OF PRESCRIBER	CAN PRESCRIBE CONTROLLED DRUGS *(SCHEDULE 2 TO 5)* ON A PRESCRIPTION.	CAN PRESCRIBE UNLICENSED MEDICINES	OTHER APPLICABLE CONSIDERATIONS	CAN AUTHORISE AN EMERGENCY SUPPLY FOR ITEMS WHICH CAN BE PRESCRIBED
DOCTOR REGISTERED IN THE UK	Yes A Home Office licence is required to prescribe cocaine, dipipanone, or diarmorphine for treating addiction Address of prescriber must be within the UK unless prescribing schedule 4 or 5 controlled drugs	Yes (subject to accepted clinical good practice)	Clinical expertise	Yes. Includes phenobarbital for epilepsy but not schedule 1,2 and 3 controlled drugs (see section 3.3.9.2)
DENTIST REGISTERED IN THE UK	Yes (but not cocaine, dipipanone or diamorphine for treating addiction) Address of prescriber must be within the UK unless prescribing schedule 4 or 5 controlled drugs	Yes (subject to accepted clinical good practice)	Should restrict prescribing to treatment of dental conditions but legally can prescribe within clinical expertise. NHS dental prescriptions are restricted to medicines within the Dental Formulary (See BNF)	Yes. Includes phenobarbital for epilepsy but not schedule 1,2 and 3 controlled drugs (see section 3.3.9.2)

UNDERPINNING KNOWLEDGE

TYPE OF PRESCRIBER	CAN PRESCRIBE CONTROLLED DRUGS *(SCHEDULE 2 TO 5)* ON A PRESCRIPTION.	CAN PRESCRIBE UNLICENSED MEDICINES	OTHER APPLICABLE CONSIDERATIONS	CAN AUTHORISE AN EMERGENCY SUPPLY FOR ITEMS WHICH CAN BE PRESCRIBED
SUPPLEMENTARY PRESCRIBER (PHARMACIST, MIDWIFE, NURSE, CHIROPODIST, PODIATRIST, PHYSIOTHERAPIST, RADIOGRAPHER OR OPTOMETRIST)	Yes (but not cocaine, dipipanone or diamorphine for treating addiction) Address of prescriber must be within the UK unless prescribing schedule 4 or 5 controlled drugs	Yes (subject to accepted clinical good practice)	Prescribed items are subject to clinical competence and inclusion within a clinical management plan agreed	Yes. Includes phenobarbital for epilepsy but not schedule 1,2 and 3 controlled drugs (see section 3.3.9.2)
NURSE INDEPENDENT PRESCRIBER	Yes (but not cocaine, dipipanone or diamorphine for treating addiction) Address of prescriber must be within the UK unless prescribing schedule 4 or 5 controlled drugs	Yes (subject to accepted clinical good practice)	Medicines for any medical condition within their competence	Yes. Includes phenobarbital for epilepsy but not schedule 1,2 and 3 controlled drugs (see section 3.3.9.2)
PHARMACIST INDEPENDENT PRESCRIBER	Yes (but not cocaine, dipipanone or diamorphine for treating addiction) Address of prescriber must be within the UK unless prescribing schedule 4 or 5 controlled drugs	Yes (subject to accepted clinical good practice)	Medicines for any medical condition within their competence	Yes. Includes phenobarbital for epilepsy but not schedule 1,2 and 3 controlled drugs (see section 3.3.9.2)
VETERINARY SURGEON AND VETERINARY PRACTITIONER	Yes (for the treatment of animals) Address of prescriber must be within the UK unless prescribing schedule 4 or 5 controlled drugs	Yes (for the treatment of animals – subject to the veterinary cascade, see section 3.6)	For the treatment of animals only	Not applicable

TYPE OF PRESCRIBER	CAN PRESCRIBE CONTROLLED DRUGS (SCHEDULE 2 TO 5) ON A PRESCRIPTION	CAN PRESCRIBE UNLICENSED MEDICINES	OTHER APPLICABLE CONSIDERATIONS	CAN AUTHORISE AN EMERGENCY SUPPLY FOR ITEMS WHICH CAN BE PRESCRIBED
EEA OR SWISS DOCTOR OR DENTIST	Schedule 4 and 5 controlled drugs only	No	Can only prescribe items which have a recognised marketing authorisation within the UK	Yes
COMMUNITY PRACTITIONER NURSE	No	No	Restricted to dressings, appliances and licensed medicines which are listed in the Nurse Prescribers' Formulary (see BNF)	Yes
OPTOMETRIST INDEPENDENT PRESCRIBER	No	No	For ocular conditions affecting the eye and surrounding tissue only	Yes

NB: Schedule 1 controlled drugs can only be prescribed under Home Office licence. Sativex holds a general licence allowing medical prescribers (doctors) to prescribe it. Non-medical prescribers are not covered by this general authority.

3.4 Wholesale dealing

As the regulatory body with responsibility for the oversight and enforcement for the wholesale of medicines, the Medicines and Healthcare products Regulatory Agency (MHRA) issued new guidance regarding the supply of medicines by pharmacy to healthcare professionals which takes effect from July 2012.

Due to the importance of supplies from pharmacies maintaining healthcare provision within the UK this guidance has been reproduced with the permission of MHRA in full below.

Regarding supplies of human medicines to veterinarians and veterinary practices for the treatment of animals please see section 3.6.

MHRA STATEMENT

Supply of medicines by pharmacy to healthcare professionals

INTRODUCTION

With effect from July 2012 Section 10(7) of the Medicines Act 1968 will be repealed. Section 10(7) currently provides an exemption in UK law from the requirement for a pharmacist to hold a Wholesale Dealer's Licence if they trade in medicines in certain circumstances. Its repeal is necessary in order to comply with EU legislation, in particular, Articles 77(1) and

77(2) of Directive 2001/83/EC which require anyone undertaking wholesale dealing activities to hold a Wholesale Dealer's Licence.

This note provides guidance for pharmacists working in registered pharmacies and in hospitals on how the MHRA, as the regulator responsible for the enforcement of EU legislation, proposes to address the implications of the necessary repeal of Section 10(7) for the supply of licensed medicines by pharmacy other than direct to the public.

THE LEGISLATION GOVERNING SUPPLY OF MEDICINES

The legislation and underpinning guidance requires persons trading in medicines to hold a Wholesale Dealer's Licence and to apply Good Distribution Practice (GDP) standards and have a suitably experienced "Responsible Person" named on the licence to ensure that medicines are procured, stored and distributed appropriately. The legislation also ensures that medicines can only be supplied to other wholesale dealers, pharmacists or other persons authorised or entitled to supply medicines to the public. These rules also serve to provide confidence in the medicines supply chain by regulating the transit of medicines from manufacturer to patient.

HOW THIS APPLIES TO SUPPLY OF MEDICINES BY PHARMACY IN THE UK

The MHRA is concerned to ensure that the repeal of the Section 10(7) exemption does not adversely impact on arrangements for supply of medicines in the UK. In determining how to address this issue, the MHRA has taken careful account of the particular arrangements for delivery of healthcare in the UK which involve a wide range of individuals and in a diverse range of locations.

In particular:

- Many healthcare professionals and others authorised or entitled to supply medicines to the public in the UK and others authorised to receive medicines, need to hold stocks of medicines for a range of purposes including local healthcare provision and look to a local community or hospital pharmacy to supply them as part of their professional practice

- In contrast, some pharmacies engage in commercial trade in medicines, not solely as part of their professional practice within the UK healthcare system

- Pharmacists may also occasionally need to obtain small quantities of a particular medicine or medicines from another pharmacist in order to meet the needs of individual patients

MHRA ENFORCEMENT

The MHRA takes the view that the supply of medicines by community and hospital pharmacies to other healthcare providers in the UK who need to hold medicines for treatment of or onward supply to their patients represents an important and appropriate part of the professional practice of both community and hospital pharmacy and falls within the definition of provision of healthcare services. In such circumstances, the MHRA will not deem such transactions as commercial dealing and pharmacies will not be required to hold a Wholesale Dealer's Licence.

Conversely, pharmacists who wish to engage in commercial trading in medicines are entitled to do so only if they hold a Wholesale Dealer's Licence and comply with all the relevant requirements. As the authority responsible for enforcement the MHRA will take appropriate action to enforce the requirement of the legislation and will require any commercial trade in medicines to be undertaken only by holders of a Wholesale Dealer's Licence.

Pharmacists needing to obtain small quantities of a medicine from another pharmacist to meet a patient's individual needs may do so without the need for the supplying pharmacy to hold a Wholesale Dealer's Licence only if the transaction meets all of the following criteria:

- It takes place on an occasional basis and

- The quantity of medicines supplied is small and intended to meet the needs of an individual patient and

- The supply is made on a not for profit basis

This restriction does not apply to exchange of stock between pharmacies that are part of the same legal entity.

Guidance on Wholesale Dealer's Licences, the application process and a downloadable application form are available on the MHRA website.

3.5 Additional legal and professional issues

3.5.1 EXPIRY DATES

Where a product states "Use by" or "Use before", this means that the product should be used before the end of the previous month. For example, "Use by 06/2011" means that the product should not be used after 31 May 2011. Although the definition of "expiry date" is less clear, the MHRA's advice to pharmaceutical manufacturers is: the term 'expiry date' should be taken to mean that the product should not be used after the end of the month stated. Therefore, an expiry date of 12/2011 means that the product should not be used after 31 December 2011.

3.5.2 WASTE MEDICINES

Information on the arrangements for disposing of pharmaceutical waste in England, Scotland and Wales is outlined in Table 3. For information regarding denaturing of controlled drugs, see section 3.7.10.

TABLE 3: WASTE ARRANGEMENTS IN ENGLAND, SCOTLAND AND WALES

For information regarding denaturing of controlled drugs, see section 3.7.10

	ENGLAND & WALES	SCOTLAND
ENFORCEMENT BODY	Environment Agency	Scottish Environment Protection Agency
CAN PHARMACIES RECEIVE WASTE MEDICINES?	Yes Generally, activities relating to waste require a licence. However, there are certain exemptions in place that allow these activities to occur without a licence. Some exemptions need to be registered while others do not. Under the Non-Waste Framework Directive (temporary storage at a collection point), pharmacies do not need to register an exemption to receive waste as long as the terms of the exemption are complied with. For further details see the Environment Agency website (**www.environment-agency.gov.uk**)	Yes The Waste Management Licensing (Scotland) Regulations 2011 allow registered pharmacies to accept returned medicines from patients or individuals and care services
SOURCES OF ADDITIONAL INFORMATION	Comprehensive information is available in a Department of Health publication entitled "Safe management of healthcare waste version 1" (**www.dh.gov.uk**) Other sources of information include the Environment Agency website (**www.environment-agency.gov.uk**) and the Pharmaceutical Services Negotiating Committee website (**www.psnc.org.uk** – information specific to England but of use in Wales)	Comprehensive information is available in a Department of Health publication "Safe management of healthcare waste version 1" (**www.dh.gov.uk**) and the Scottish Health Technical Note 3 Part B – NHS Scotland Waste Management Guidance: Waste Management Policy Template (**www.hfs.scot.nhs.uk**) Other sources of information include the Scottish Environment Protection Agency website (**www.sepa.org.uk**)
WHERE SHOULD WASTE MEDICINES BE STORED?	Waste medicines must be kept in secure waste containers in a designated area preferably away from medicines that are fit for use. If sharps are accepted, they should be stored in a sharps container	
DEALING WITH CONFIDENTIAL INFORMATION	Ensure that any patient identifiable information is destroyed or totally obscured	
TABLETS AND CAPSULES	Blister strips can be removed from their inert outer packaging but tablets should not be de-blistered. *(NB: An exemption applies to controlled drug tablets and capsules, which require denaturing – see section 3.7.10)*	

	ENGLAND & WALES	SCOTLAND
SHARPS	Dispose of syringes and needles in a sharps container.	
LIQUIDS	The whole bottle (including empty bottles that may contain residue) should be placed into a pharmaceutical waste container because the mixing of different medicines could be hazardous. *(NB: Exceptions apply to controlled drug liquids, which require denaturing – see section 3.7.10)*	
ADVICE FOR PATIENTS	Patients should be advised that unused, unwanted medicines should be returned to a pharmacy for safe disposal	

3.5.3 COSMETIC CONTACT LENSES (ZERO POWERED)

Pharmacists who intend to sell cosmetic contact lenses (zero powered) need to consider the legal requirements within the Opticians Act 1989 and any subsequent rules and regulations that control the sale of such contact lenses. These products can only be sold under the supervision of a registered optician, dispensing optician or doctor.

FURTHER INFORMATION

The General Optical Council can be consulted on 0207 580 3898 (**www.optical.org**)

3.5.4 REQUESTS FOR CHEMICALS

Traditionally, a pharmacist's role included the supply of a range of chemicals. However, most modern pharmacists focus more on supplying medicinal products to patients safely and responsibly. Consequently, the retail sale of chemicals for non-medicinal purposes is no longer a core role for a pharmacist.

It is within this context that pharmacists should consider the following before making a judgment on the retail sale of chemicals:

- Who is requesting the chemical and are they known to the pharmacy?
- What is being requested?
- How much is being requested?
- What is the purpose of the purchase?
- Does the purpose of the purchase mean that there are likely to be additional legal implications?
- Is the pharmacy the most appropriate place to obtain the chemical?
- Are there more appropriate commercial alternatives to the product being requested?

- Is there any suspicion of inappropriate or illicit use and does a "Chemical suspicious activity report" need to be submitted to the Serious Organised Crime Agency?

In addition, packaging and labelling regulations for chemicals (also known as 'CHIP regulations') and Control of Substances Hazardous to Health (COSHH) regulations should be considered.

FURTHER RESOURCES

Online resources on CHIP and COSHH regulations are available on the Health and Safety Executive website (**www.hse.gov.uk**)

Chemical suspicious activity report resources are available on the Serious Organised Crime Agency website (**www.soca.gov.uk**)

3.5.5 DELIVERY AND POSTING OF MEDICINES TO PATIENTS *(INCLUDING ABROAD)*

There are professional and practical considerations that are important when deciding whether or not to deliver medicines or whether or not to post medicines (prescribed or sold) to patients. The following are important to consider when making a professional judgment: (The list is not exhaustive)

- Patient consent for delivery or posting
- Patient confidentiality during the delivery or posting process
- Whether it is necessary for face-to-face contact with the patient to ensure that the medicine can be safely, effectively and appropriately used
- Whether it is necessary to interview the patient
- Whether the patient has been assessed or directly interviewed by the prescriber
- An adequate audit trail for delivery and receipt from the point at which the medicine leaves the pharmacy and is received by the patient (or returned to the pharmacy in the event of delivery failure)
- Storage requirements during transit
- When posting – will the postal carrier agree to transport the medicinal product (check terms of carriage, prohibited and restricted goods)

- When posting abroad – are there legal restrictions in the destination country which would prevent you from posting? (As an example, guidance produced by the U.S. Food and Drug Administration (FDA) makes it clear that it is illegal or a foreign pharmacy to ship prescription medicines that are not approved by the FDA to the United States)
- When posting abroad – are there UK legal restrictions which would prevent you dispensing in the first instance? (e.g. is the prescriber recognised as an appropriate practitioner (see 3.3.1) for the medicinal product in the UK?)

FURTHER RESOURCES

Lists of internationally recognised narcotic and psychotropic drugs are available on the International Narcotics Control Board website (**www.incb.org**).

United States Food and Drug Administration (FDA). Buying medicines and medicinal products online FAQs (available under Drugs tab, resources for consumers **www.fda.gov**)

3.5.6 SECURE ENVIRONMENTS

Secure environments include prisons, police custody suites, secure hospitals, immigration removal centres, and other places where persons are detained. Medicines and other health legislation may not refer specifically to the particular environment, and where this is the case then consideration should be given to best practice in either primary or secondary care, as appropriate, acting within the confines of the relevant legislation.

When medicines are dispensed from an 'in-house' pharmacy for administration or supply to patients within a prison, the pharmacy does not need to be registered with the General Pharmaceutical Council. Nonetheless, general pharmaceutical legal and good practice guidelines should be followed. If provision of a pharmacy service to another prison is being considered from an in-house pharmacy, advice should be obtained from the GPhC and MHRA to discuss whether the pharmacy premises would require registration or whether a wholesale dealer's licence will be required.

The Secure Environment Pharmacists Group (SEPG) is a special interest group for pharmacists directly providing professional pharmacy and/or medicines management services to prisons or other secure environments. The SEPG provides an opportunity for networking and peer-level support and for the sharing of good practice.

FURTHER RESOURCES

Further information and resources for pharmacists working in secure environments can be found on the SEPG virtual network – accessible from the RPS website (**www.rpharms.com**)

3.5.7 CHECKING REGISTRATION OF HEALTHCARE PROFESSIONALS

Pharmacists may need to verify the registration status of other pharmacists and other healthcare professionals as part of the due diligence process when checking whether a person can prescribe or whether they can be wholesaled to.

Table 4 provides details on where registration information can be verified (along with additional relevant notes) for several types of healthcare professional.

TABLE 4: HOW TO CHECK REGISTRATION FOR HEALTHCARE PROFESSIONALS

HEALTHCARE PROFESSIONAL	WHERE TO CHECK REGISTRATION	COMMON ISSUES
PHARMACISTS	General Pharmaceutical Council (**www.pharmacyregulation.org**) 020 3365 3400	There are pharmacists with further qualifications, such as independent or supplementary prescribers, and this is reflected in the register Supplementary prescribers can prescribe all medicines included in a clinical management plan agreed with a prescriber and the patient. This includes controlled drugs and unlicensed medicines Independent prescribers can prescribe unlicensed medicines and since 23 April 2012 have also been able to prescribe controlled drugs. Prescribing should be restricted to areas of clinical competence Further information on non-medical prescribing, including FAQs, guidance and clinical management plans is available on the Department of Health website (**www.dh.gov.uk**)
PHARMACY TECHNICIANS	General Pharmaceutical Council (**www.pharmacyregulation.org**) 020 3365 3400	
DOCTORS	General Medical Council (**www.gmc-uk.org**) 0161 923 6602	To practise medicine in the UK, doctors are required to be registered with the GMC and hold a licence to practise
DENTISTS	General Dental Council (**www.gdc-uk.org**) 0845 222 4141	Dentists can legally write prescriptions for any medicine but they should restrict their prescribing to areas in which they are competent. Therefore they should, generally, only prescribe medicines that have uses in dentistry When prescribing on an NHS dental prescription, dentists are restricted to the medicines listed in the Dental Practitioners' Formulary (part 8a of the Drug Tariff for Scotland or part XVIIa of the Drug Tariff for England and Wales)

HEALTHCARE PROFESSIONAL	WHERE TO CHECK REGISTRATION	COMMON ISSUES
NURSES	Nursing and Midwifery Council (**www.nmc-uk.org**) 020 7333 9333	Nurses can have a range of further qualifications, which are annotated on the NMC register. Prescribing should be restricted to areas of clinical competence Further information on non-medical prescribing, including FAQs, guidance and clinical management plans is available on the Department of Health website (**www.dh.gov.uk**)
VETERINARY SURGEONS	Royal College of Veterinary Surgeons (**www.rcvs.org.uk**) 020 7222 2001	Veterinary surgeons can prescribe and requisition all human and animal medicines, including controlled drugs for the treatment of animals. Where controlled drugs are involved, these do not need to be on standardised forms Where the medicine is not licensed for the animal, then this needs to be prescribed under the veterinary cascade (see section for further details)
PARAMEDICS	Health Professions Council (**www.hpc-uk.org**) 020 7582 0866	A Home Office group authority has been issued that allows paramedics to possess and supply certain controlled drugs under certain conditions. The Home Office has the authority to revoke or modify the authority at any time A full list of medicines that a paramedic can obtain for the purposes of administration is available on the MHRA website (**www.mhra.gov.uk**)
CHIROPODISTS OR PODIATRISTS	Health Professions Council (**www.hpc-uk.org**) 020 7582 0866	Registered chiropodists and podiatrists can obtain additional qualifications that allow them to sell or supply and administer a larger range of medicines A full list of medicines that a chiropodist can sell, supply or administer is available on the MHRA website (**www.mhra.gov.uk**)
PHYSIOTHERAPISTS	Health Professions Council (**www.hpc-uk.org**) 020 7582 0866	

UNDERPINNING KNOWLEDGE

HEALTHCARE PROFESSIONAL	WHERE TO CHECK REGISTRATION	COMMON ISSUES
OPTOMETRISTS	General Optical Council (**www.optical.org**) 020 7580 3898	Optometrists can take further qualifications to become an "additional supply optometrist" – this increases the range of medicines that they can sell or supply to patients (and therefore obtain by wholesale from a pharmacy). A full list of the medicines that can be obtained is available from the MHRA website (**www.mhra.gov.uk**) Further information on non-medical prescribing, including FAQs, guidance and clinical management plans is available on the Department of Health website (**www.dh.gov.uk**)

3.5.8 CHILD-RESISTANT CONTAINERS

Suitable, re-closable child-resistant containers (CRCs) should be used for supplying all solid and all oral and external liquid dose preparations unless there is a good reason for not doing so. Such reasons may include:

- **SPECIFIC REQUEST** – the patient, carer or representative requests a container that is not child resistant, perhaps due to difficulty in opening a CRC. The request may be met by supplying a non-CRC lid

- **ORIGINAL PACK** – the original pack may not be child resistant and there may be reasons underpinning why the medicine should remain in the original container. It may also be the case that no CRC exists for a particular liquid medicine so it is not possible to change the container

Where appropriate, the patient should be counselled to keep medicines away from the reach and sight of children.

3.5.9 REPORTING ADVERSE EVENTS

The role of most pharmacists involves contact with patients and receiving information from patients. Consequently they are in a prime position to identify adverse drug reactions. The Royal Pharmaceutical Society encourages, as a matter of best practice, the reporting of suspected adverse drug reactions under the Yellow Card scheme. Following a discussion with the patient, it may also be appropriate to make a record in the patient's notes and to notify the prescriber.

Reporting is possible online at **www.yellowcard.gov.uk**. Otherwise, a tear-out paper copy is available at the back of the BNF.

If a suspected adverse drug reaction (SADR) is related to a veterinary medicine which has affected a human and/or an animal, refer to section 3.6.

3.5.10 EMERGENCY CONNECTION TO EX-DIRECTORY TELEPHONE NUMBERS

Pharmacists can be connected to ex-directory, no-connection telephone numbers if they need to contact patients in a real emergency. This privilege is also available to doctors, hospitals and emergency authorities.

Pharmacists must use the privilege appropriately and only exercise their right of access when strictly necessary. The following guidelines must be adhered to:

- Pharmacists should only consider asking for connection to an ex-directory, no-connection number in a life or death situation. This can be interpreted as an emergency that is likely to pose a very serious threat to the health of a patient if information cannot be passed on immediately and when the patient's telephone number cannot be found from another source (e.g. the patient's GP surgery)

- A pharmacist needing to contact an ex-directory, no-connection number should dial 100, explain the situation and request connection to the number
- The pharmacist will only be connected when the following criteria are met:
  - the pharmacist explains the reason for the emergency connection request and advises the operator that it is a life or death situation (the operator will not judge the nature of the emergency but will accept the word of the pharmacist)
  - the pharmacist must give his or her name and the name of the pharmacy premises from which he or she is calling

BT monitors all requests for emergency connection. If the privilege is abused it is likely that this important facility will be withdrawn.

3.5.11 HOMEOPATHIC AND HERBAL REMEDIES

Homeopathy has been defined as a holistic complementary and alternative therapy based on the concept of like to treat like and involves the administration of dilute and ultradilute products prepared according to methods given in homeopathic pharmacopoeias.

Herbal preparations contain plant-derived materials, either as raw or processed ingredients which may be from one or more plants.

DIFFERENCES BETWEEN HOMEOPATHIC AND HERBAL PRODUCTS

The public can confuse homeopathic with herbal products as homeopathic products are often derived from herbs and are called by their botanical name, e.g. aloe, and also because a single manufacturer may produce both homeopathic and herbal products. Pharmacists can help the public understand the difference between homeopathy and herbal products using information in our comparison table.

TABLE 5: COMPARISON OF HOMEOPATHIC AND HERBAL PRODUCTS

	HOMEOPATHIC PRODUCTS	HERBAL PRODUCTS
WHAT ARE THEY MADE FROM?	Often plants but may be from mineral, animal or even synthetic material	Naturally occurring plants, parts of plants or extracts of plants
DO THEY CONTAIN ACTIVE INGREDIENTS?	Generally the starting material is diluted so that few or no molecules of the starting material remain in the product. Some products are administered orally and topically that do contain measurable amounts of the starting material and such products are deemed to be homeopathic because of their method of preparation	Often contain mixtures of many chemical compounds obtained from the plant although precise compositions can be variable due to the natural source
HOW IS THE PRODUCT MADE?	Homeopaths believe that serial dilution and succussion (shaking) steps are critical in ensuring the efficacy of the product. They believe that the more succussion that takes place through the dilution steps, the more energy is imparted and the more efficacious the product	Herbal products are prepared using either extracts of the herbal material or the crude drug itself

	HOMEOPATHIC PRODUCTS	HERBAL PRODUCTS
HOW ARE PRODUCTS SELECTED?	Homeopaths believe in the three principles of homeopathy, one of which is that like should be treated with like. For example, they believe that a substance that causes vomiting in high doses may be used to treat vomiting using a very dilute product	In a manner similar to other medicines, herbal products are selected according to the range of symptoms they are known to treat. They are often used to restore, correct or modify a physiological function
HOW IS A PARTICULAR PRODUCT SELECTED?	Homeopathic practitioners adopt a holistic approach where a detailed patient consultation takes place prior to a suitable product being recommended. The self selection of homeopathic products is typically based on their traditional use in homeopathy	Based on the symptoms presented, a product is selected taking account of the known pharmacological activity of the herbal product
HOW DOES THE DOES EFFECT THE EFFICACY OF THE PRODUCT?	Due to extensive dilution, homeopathy usually involves the administration of none, or an incredibly small amount, of the starting material. Homeopaths believe that the greater the dilution of a product the more potent and efficacious it becomes	Increasing the dose will increase the effect and/or increase the risk of adverse effects
ARE THE PRODUCTS SAFE?	Generally considered by homeopaths to be non-toxic and safe for administration to adults and children, particularly at high dilution. It is important to note that not all homeopathic products are not ultradilute and may contain discernible amounts of the starting material. (*see footnote)	Although they are obtained from natural sources, they are not without unwanted effects and cannot be regarded as safe. The active substance in many prescription medicines is obtained or derived from plant sources
ARE THERE ANY SIDE EFFECTS?	Side effects have not been reported in the scientific literature for high dilution products. Homeopaths believe homeopathic products can cause aggravations (exacerbations or worsening of symptoms). May cause reactions in lactose intolerant patients. (*see footnote)	May produce side effects
WILL THEY INTERACT WITH PRESCRIPTION OR OTHER MEDICINES?	No evidence of interactions between high dilution products and conventional medicines. (*see footnote)	Can interact with prescription and other conventional medicines
ARE THEY SAFE IN PREGNANCY AND WHEN BREASTFEEDING?	Considered by homeopaths to be suitable for use during pregnancy and while breastfeeding, but ideally under the guidance of a suitably qualified homeopath. However it is important that patients inform healthcare professionals if they are taking a homeopathic product during pregnancy and while breastfeeding, even if it is a highly diluted product. (*see footnote)	Certain herbal ingredients should be avoided or used with caution in pregnancy and while breastfeeding

	HOMEOPATHIC PRODUCTS	HERBAL PRODUCTS
SHOULD I INFORM OTHER HEALTHCARE PROFESSIONALS IF I AM TAKING THESE PRODUCTS?	Although homeopaths believe this is not necessary, it is important that patients inform healthcare professionals if they are taking a homeopathic product, even if it is highly diluted. (*see footnote)	Patients should inform healthcare professionals if they are taking herbal products
LABELLING	Will include the words "homeopathic medicinal product" on the label	Licensed herbal medicines will include a product licence (PL) number. Those products registered under the Traditional Herbal Medicines Registration Scheme will include a statement to the effect that it is a traditional herbal medicinal product for use in specified indication(s) exclusively based on long standing use. The packaging will also have a THR number and may include the THR certification mark
IS IT KNOWN HOW THEY WORK?	There is no sound scientific basis to explain the activity of homeopathic products claimed by homeopaths	The effects of the active ingredients in a herbal product can be shown to have pharmacological actions
WHAT IS THE EVIDENCE TO SUPPORT THE EFFICACY OF THESE PRODUCTS?	There is no scientific or clinical evidence to support the efficacy of homeopathic products above the placebo effect, although anecdotal reports of their effectiveness have been published, particularly when used as part of individualised homeopathic treatment by a homeopathic practitioner	There is scientific evidence to support the efficacy of a limited number of herbal products in specific conditions; however, for many herbal products, efficacy has not been formally evaluated using the same randomised clinical trials as routinely used for licensed medicines

* Mother tinctures or homeopathic products of low dilution will contain measurable amounts of active materials. For those homeopathic products, it is more appropriate to use the guidance given for herbal products.

EVIDENCE FOR HOMEOPATHY

There is no scientific or clinical evidence to support the efficacy of homeopathic products above the placebo effect, although anecdotal reports of their effectiveness have been published, particularly when used as part of individualised homeopathic treatment by a homeopathic practitioner. There is no evidence to support the clinical efficacy of homeopathic products beyond a placebo effect, and no scientific basis for homeopathy.

Given the lack of clinical and scientific evidence to support homeopathy, the RPS does not endorse homeopathy as a form of treatment.

ADVICE FOR PATIENTS

If a patient requests advice on homeopathy, the pharmacist should advise on the lack of evidence on the efficacy of homeopathic products, discuss the formulation and composition of the product, and provide advice relevant to the patient's condition. Pharmacists should also ensure that patients do not stop taking their prescribed medication if they take a homeopathic product.

REFERRAL

Pharmacists will be in a position to identify serious, underlying undiagnosed medical conditions requiring the patients to be referred to another healthcare professional.

UNDERPINNING KNOWLEDGE

Homeopathic products should only be used for the treatment of minor, self-limiting conditions, and must never be used for the treatment of serious medical conditions.

LICENSING

For the purpose of licensing, the MHRA does not currently require homeopathic products to demonstrate efficacy, only quality and safety. Further information about regulation of homeopathic products and registration is available on the MHRA website (**www.mhra.gov.uk**). Herbal remedies must either have a full marketing authorisation based upon safety, quality and efficacy or a traditional herbal registration (THR) based upon safety, quality and evidence of traditional use. Further information is available on the MHRA website (**www.mhra.gov.uk**).

FURTHER RESOURCES

RPS Support. *Homeopathic and herbal products – quick reference guide.* February 2010. (**www.rpharms.com**)

RPS Support. *The traditional registration scheme – quick reference guide.* (**www.rpharms.com**)

Williamson E, Driver S, Baxter K. *Stockley's Herbal Medicines Interactions,* London: Pharmaceutical Press, 2009.

Barnes J, Anderson L, Phillipson J. *Herbal Medicines 3rd Edition,* London: Pharmaceutical Press 2007

3.5.12 CHARITABLE DONATIONS

The World Health Organization in co-operation with major international agencies involved with humanitarian and developmental aid (including the International Pharmaceutical Federation (FIP), International Federation of the Red Cross and Red Crescent Societies) has published guidance (first edition 1996) that provides clear guidelines for the donation of medicine. We encourage any pharmacist considering donating medicines to read the document and adhere to the guidelines.

CONSIDER ALTERNATIVES

WHO encourages, in the acute phase of an emergency, that standardised health kits of medicines are donated. These kits are permanently stocked by major international suppliers such as Médecins Sans Frontières and the United Nations Children's Fund.

After the acute phase, WHO encourages the donation of cash that can be used to purchase essential medicines and is usually more useful than donations of drugs.

PATIENT RETURNS

There are ethical arguments for and against donating patient returns. However, it should be noted that the WHO guidelines specifically advise that patient returns should not be donated.

REFERENCES

World Health Organization. *Guidelines for medicines donations* (3rd edition). Revised 2010. (**www.who.int**)

3.5.13 ELECTRONIC CIGARETTE (INTERIM ADVICE)

Electronic cigarettes resemble cigarettes and deliver nicotine to the user via inhalation.

These articles are currently not medicinal products; they do not hold marketing authorisations as medicinal products and are not intended for nicotine replacement therapy (NRT) or smoking cessation.

Licensed NRT medicines which hold marketing authorisations exist in a range of formulations, including as a non-electronic inhalator product.

Medicines which hold marketing authorisations benefit from assurance of quality, safety, efficacy, and from processes underpinned by Good Manufacturing Practice (GMP).

Articles that do not have marketing authorisations do not benefit from the same quality control processes.

While these products remain unregulated, there is a gap in scientific evidence in terms of quality, safety and efficacy compared with medicinal products and devices, and the Royal Pharmaceutical Society therefore does not endorse the use of electronic cigarettes as a form of treatment.

The involvement of community pharmacists and pharmacy staff in the sale of these articles alongside licensed NRT may provide a mistaken impression of legitimacy that electronic cigarettes are equivalent to proven medicinal products or medical devices when they are not.

This, together with the gap in evidence, could mean that sales by pharmacists are not in patients' best interests.

FURTHER INFORMATION

European Commission Orientation note, Electronic cigarettes and the EC legislation (May 2008) European Commission website

U.S. Food and Drug Administration *Online public health news, Electronic Cigarettes* (**www.fda.gov**)

World Health Organisation *Online news release, Marketers of electronic cigarettes should halt unproved therapy claims* (**www.who.int**)

3.5.14 SOCIAL MEDIA

Pharmacists and aspiring pharmacists who use social media* and social networking* should do so responsibly and with the same high standards which they would apply in real–world interactions.

In particular, it is important to maintain proper professional boundaries in relationships and interactions with patients and at all times to respect the confidentiality of others, including patients and colleagues.

Be aware of the potential audience of your online activity, and that this may be publicly accessible, circulated and shared beyond your control. This activity could impact upon your professional image and the reputation of the profession as a whole.

Remember that General Pharmaceutical Council (GPhC) standards of conduct, ethics and performance (see Appendix 1) include standard and which require pharmacists to:

Treat people politely and considerately

AND

Maintain proper professional boundaries in your relationships with patients and others that you come into contact with during the course of your professional practice and take special care when dealing with vulnerable people.

These standards would apply in the real world as well as with social media*.

Social media includes blogging, web forums including professional web forums, Twitter, Facebook, online and virtual networks (this list is not exhaustive).

3.5.15 COLLECTION OF MEDICINE BY CHILDREN

Pharmacists may be asked to supply dispensed medicines to a child for themselves or on behalf of another person, such as a parent, other relative or neighbour.

The decision on whether a supply is appropriate will need to be dealt with on a case by case basis and will involve considering the individual circumstances. Sometimes there will not be a clear right or wrong decision, and different pharmacists with the same facts will make different choices. Whatever your decision, you should be prepared to justify this and make records of decisions where appropriate.

If in doubt, the following are some of the factors the pharmacist may want to consider, when deciding whether the supply of the dispensed medicines is appropriate or not. It is not possible for this list to be exhaustive.

1. **KNOWLEDGE OF THE CHILD:** Is the child known to the pharmacy? What information is known?

2. **MATURITY OF THE CHILD:** Is the pharmacist satisfied the child is capable and competent to understand the importance of the medicines they are collecting and are you satisfied there are no further concerns with them delivering the medicines. If the medicine is prescribed for the child, and the child is competent then patient confidentiality applies (see Appendix 4).

3. **NATURE OF THE MEDICINE(S) SUPPLIED:** What are

the medicines being collected? Is there any applicable misuse potential? Is the pharmacist confident the child will not misuse or tamper with the medicine?

4. **PRIOR ARRANGEMENT:** Does the child regularly collect medicines from the pharmacy? Is the collection by the child pre-arranged by the patient? For example, an advance phone call by the patient or a letter of explanation.

5. **REASON FOR COLLECTION:** Is there a persuasive reason behind why the child is collecting the medicine in the circumstances? For example, is collection on behalf of a patient who has mobility problems or is the child expected to self-medicate such as with an inhaler.

6. **COUNSELLING:** Does the patient require counselling? How will this be given? If the patient is the child, are they able to understand?

7. **LOCAL POLICIES:** Are there any local policies which you should consider in your pharmacy or your local area?

8. **PROOF OF IDENTITY:** In some circumstances, such as with the supply of schedule 2 controlled drugs, the pharmacist will usually ask to see identification of the collecting patient or representative. Children may not have ID to show and professional judgment can be used to decide if a supply is appropriate without identification.

3.6 Veterinary medicines

Pharmacists working in registered premises are authorised to supply veterinary medicines for use in animals under certain circumstances (e.g. when there is a valid prescription) and, as with human medicines, are responsible for any medicines supplied. There are various classes of veterinary medicines, which are summarised in Table 6.

TABLE 6: CATEGORIES OF VETERINARY MEDICINES AND THEIR CHARACTERISTIC

POM-V	Prescription-only medicines that can only be prescribed by a veterinary surgeon and supplied by a veterinary surgeon or a pharmacist with a written prescription
POM-VPS	Prescription-only medicines that can be prescribed and supplied by a veterinary surgeon, a pharmacist or a suitably qualified person on an oral or written prescription. A written prescription is only required if the supplier is not the prescriber
NFA-VPS	A category of medicine for non-food animals that can be supplied by a veterinary surgeon, a pharmacist or a suitably qualified person. A written prescription is not required
AVM-GSL	An authorised veterinary medicine that is available on general sale
EXEMPT MEDICINES UNDER THE SMALL ANIMAL EXEMPTION SCHEME (SAES)	An unlicensed veterinary medicine that does not require a marketing authorisation because it meets criteria laid out in the SAES. Further details are available from the Veterinary Medicines Directorate website (**www.vmd.defra.gov.uk**)
UNAUTHORISED VETERINARY MEDICINE	An unlicensed medicine that does not have a marketing authorisation and is not eligible for exemption through the SAES. It can only be prescribed by a veterinary surgeon under the cascade (see below). This includes any human medicine used for animals

Prescription requirements for POM-V, POM-VPS and medicines supplied under the veterinary cascade

The following must be present for a veterinary medicine prescription to be valid:

1. Name, address, telephone number, qualification and signature of the prescriber

2. Name and address of the owner

3. Identification and species of the animal and its address (if different from the owner's address)

❶ P NIGHTINGALE MRCVS
PRACTICE NAME,
ADDRESS,
TOWN,
POSTCODE
TEL: 0202 33 22 44 55

Endorsements

❸ PRESCRIPTION FOR SPOT THE DALMATIAN

❷ OWNED BY MRS R SWANN OF
ADDRESS, TOWN, POSTCODE

❺ SUPPLY PHENYTOIN SODIUM CAPSULES 100MG X 90
5 CAPSULES 3 TIMES A DAY WITH FOOD
❻

❾ REPEAT X 4

❼ PRESCRIBED UNDER THE VETERINARY CASCADE

Signature of Prescriber | Date
❶ P. Nightingale | **❹** 30TH JULY 2012

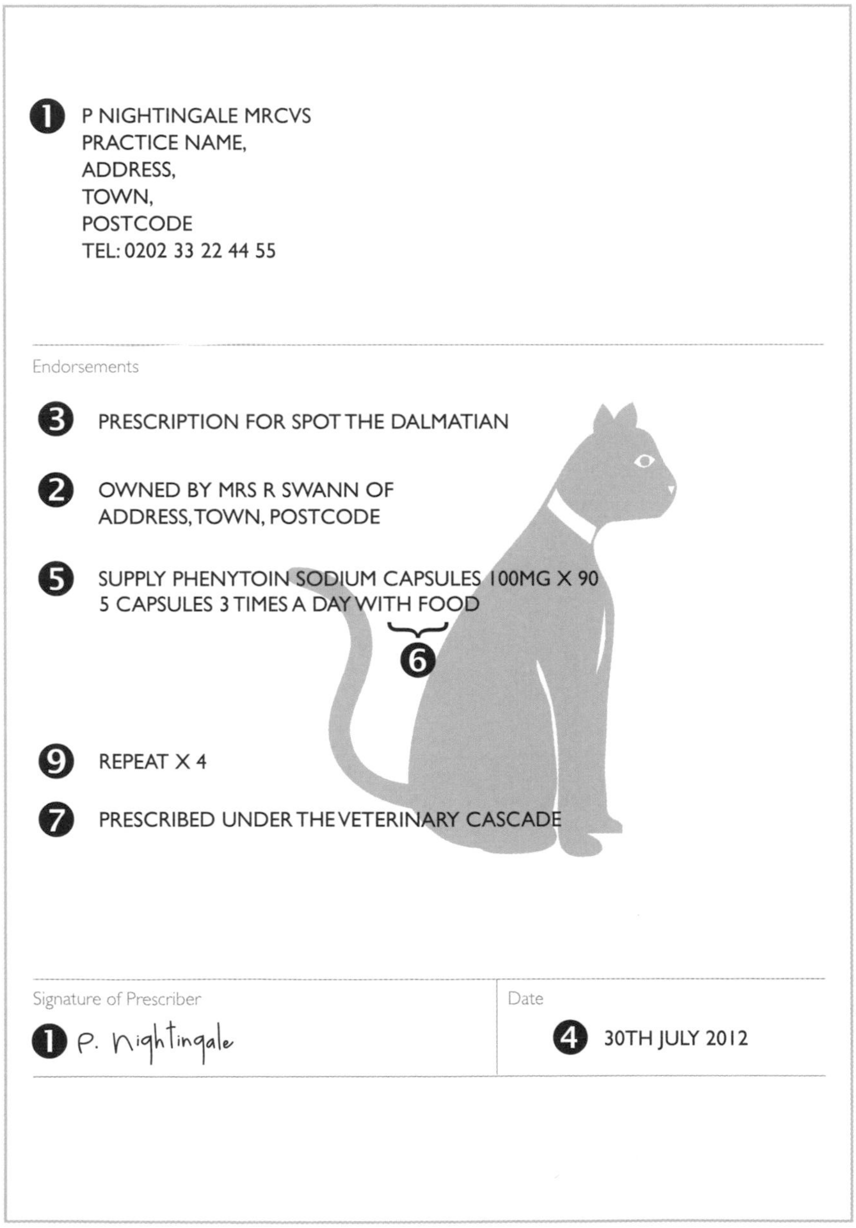

DIAGRAM 4: VETERINARY PRESCRIPTION WITH CASCADE WORDING

4. Date; prescriptions are valid for six months or shorter if indicated by the prescriber. Prescriptions for schedule 2, 3 and 4 controlled drugs are valid for 28 days

5. Name, quantity, dose and administration instructions of the required medicine
NB: The Veterinary Medicines Directorate advises that "as directed" is not an acceptable administration instruction

6. Any necessary warnings and if relevant the withdrawal period (i.e. the time that must elapse between when an animal receives a medicine and when it can be used for food)

7. Where appropriate, a statement highlighting that the medicine is prescribed under the veterinary cascade (e.g. "prescribed under the cascade" or other wording to the same effect)

8. Where schedule 2 or 3 controlled drugs have been prescribed, a declaration that "the item has been prescribed for an animal or herd under the care of the veterinarian" – usual controlled drugs prescription requirements apply (see section 3.7.7)

9. If the prescription is repeatable, the number of times it can be repeated

TABLE 7: SIMILARITIES AND DIFFERENCES BETWEEN VETERINARY AND HUMAN CONTROLLED DRUG PRESCRIPTIONS

DIFFERENCES BETWEEN HUMAN AND VETERINARY PRESCRIPTIONS	SIMILARITIES BETWEEN HUMAN AND VETERINARY PRESCRIPTIONS
Standardised forms are not required for veterinary prescriptions, however a statement that the medicines are "prescribed for the treatment of an animal or herd under my care" is required. Veterinary prescriptions should be retained for five years and not submitted to the relevant NHS agency.	Both are valid for 28 days from the appropriate date. Repeatable prescriptions (e.g. repeat x 3) are not acceptable for either type of prescription for schedule 2 and 3 controlled drugs. Usual controlled drug prescription content requirements (e.g. total quantity in words and figures, etc – see section 3.7.7) apply to both.

The veterinary cascade

A veterinary medicine with a UK marketing authorisation must be prescribed and supplied where one exists and is clinically appropriate. The cascade exemption within the Veterinary Medicines Regulations allows the supply of medicines that are not licensed for animals. It is unlawful to supply a human medicine against a veterinary prescription unless it is prescribed by a veterinary surgeon and specifically states that it is "for administration under the cascade", or other wording to this effect. The Veterinary Medicines Directorate (VMD) has issued guidance which requires the veterinary surgeon to use their judgment to list the safety warnings that should be incorporated onto the label of the dispensed cascade medicine.

NB: Although the wording on the prescription is a legal requirement, it is important that it reflects the actual cascade (i.e. if a prescription is written generically for an animal with the cascade wording present but a licensed veterinary medicine exists, then the cascade requires the licensed product to be supplied rather than a medicine only licensed for human use).

The exemption specifies that where a licensed veterinary product is not available, other medicines can be considered as shown in diagram 5.

Veterinary medicines licensed for another species, or for another clinical condition in the same species, extemporaneously prepared medicines or human medicines cannot be supplied against a veterinary prescription unless the prescription specifically states that it is "for administration under the cascade", or other wording to this effect.

Where available it is a legal requirement to:

Supply a licensed veterinary medicine

Only where the above is not possible:

An existing licensed veterinary medicine for another species or different condition can be considered

Only where the above is not possible:

A licensed human medicine or an EU-licensed veterinary medicine can be considered

Only where the above is not possible:

Extemporaneous or specially manufactured medicines can be considered

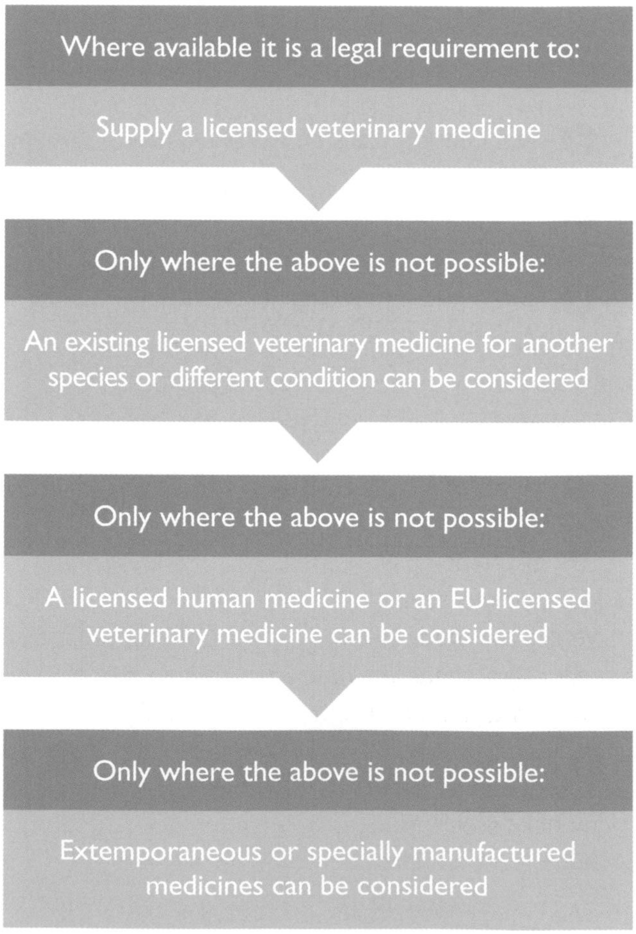

DIAGRAM 5: VETERINARY CASCADE

Labelling

When a medicine is supplied by a pharmacy for use under the cascade, the following details must appear on the dispensing label unless they already appear on the packaging and are not obscured by the dispensing label:

- Name of the prescribing veterinary surgeon
- Name and address of the animal owner
- Name and address of the pharmacy
- Identification and species of the animal
- Date of supply
- Expiry date of the product
- The name or description of the product or its active ingredients and content quantity
- Dosage and administration instructions
- If appropriate, special storage instructions
- Any necessary warnings for the user (e.g. relating to administration, disposal, target species, etc)
- Any applicable withdrawal period (i.e. the time between when an animal receives a medicine and when it can safely be used for food)
- The words: "For animal treatment only"
- The words: "Keep out of reach of children"

If the medicine is not prescribed under the cascade, the Veterinary Medicines Regulations do not specify that a dispensing label is required. However, the Royal Pharmaceutical Society advises that it would be appropriate to generate a dispensing label for all veterinary medicines, particularly for individual animals (pets).

Record keeping

The following points should be considered regarding record keeping for veterinary medicines:

- Records must be kept for receipts and supplies of POM-V and POM-VPS products and must show:
  - name of the medicine
  - date of the receipt or supply
  - batch number
  - quantity
  - name and address of the supplier or recipient
- If there is a written prescription, record the name and address of the prescriber and keep a copy of the prescription
- Pharmacists can either keep all documents that show the required information or can make appropriate records in their private prescription book
- Records can be kept electronically
- Records and documents must be kept for at least five years
- Pharmacies that supply POM-V and POM-VPS medicines must undertake an annual audit

---

SALE OF UNAUTHORISED VETERINARY MEDICINES

It is unlawful to sell or supply unauthorised veterinary medicines (medicines not licensed as veterinary medicines), including human medicines such as GSL and P medicines, for an animal unless this takes place under the veterinary cascade. This applies even if a veterinary surgeon asks the animal owner verbally to purchase an over-the-counter human product from a pharmacy.

SALE OF NFA-VPS AND POM-VPS MEDICINES

It is a legal requirement for pharmacists who supply NFA-VPS medicines or prescribe POM-VPS medicines to:

- Advise on how to use the product safely
- Advise on any applicable warnings and contra-indications on the packaging or label
- Be satisfied that the recipient intends to use the medicine correctly and is competent to do so
- Prescribe or supply the minimum quantity required for treatment

PHYSICAL PRESENCE OF A PHARMACIST

Unless a transaction has been individually authorised in advance by a pharmacist and the person handing out the medicine is judged to be competent, the physical presence of the pharmacist is required for POM-V, POM-VPS and NFA-VPS medicines to be supplied.

ADVERSE REACTIONS

Pharmacists are increasingly supplying veterinary medicines for companion animals and should be mindful to the possibility that veterinary medicines can cause adverse reactions in humans as well as in animals exposed to a veterinary medicine. Suspect adverse drug reactions (SADRs) in humans are often associated with a failure to read and/or adequately follow product guidance information. Examples include animal sprays and 'spot-ons' onto human skin.

The adverse reaction scheme for veterinary medicines is the equivalent of the 'yellow card' scheme for human medicines. Both animal adverse reactions and human adverse reactions to veterinary medicinal products should be reported. Details of the scheme and reporting forms are available on the VMD website (**www.vmd.defra.gov.uk/adversereactionreporting**) or directly from VMD on 01932 338427.

FURTHER READING

The Veterinary Pharmacy Forum virtual network is available to members on the RPS website (**www.rpharms.com**)

Online resources, including a database of veterinary medicinal products and guidance documents are available on the Veterinary Medicines Directorate website (**www.vmd.defra.gov.uk**)

Veterinary Medicines Directorate. *Veterinary medicines advice for pharmacists leaflet 2012* (**www.vmd.defra.gov.uk**)

National Office of Animal Health. *NOAH compendium of data sheets for animal medicines.* 2011. (**www.noahcompendium.co.uk**)

Details of a formal post-graduate veterinary pharmacy programme are available from the Harper Adams University College website (**www.harper-adams.ac.uk**)

Kayne S. *An Introduction to Veterinary Medicine;* Saltire Books; 2011

3.7 Controlled drugs

3.7.1 BACKGROUND

The core pieces of pharmacy legislation applicable to controlled drugs are:

- The Misuse of Drugs Act 1971 as amended (herein referred to as "the 1971 Act")
- The Misuse of Drugs Regulations 2001 as amended (herein referred to as "the 2001 Regulations")
- The Misuse of Drugs (Safe Custody) Regulations 1973 as amended (herein referred to as "Safe Custody Regulations")
- The Health Act 2006

The 1971 Act imposes prohibitions on the possession, supply, manufacture, import and export of controlled drugs – except where permitted by the 2001 Regulations or under licence from the Secretary of State. The Safe Custody Regulations detail the storage and safe custody requirements for controlled drugs. The enforcement body for controlled drug offences is the Home Office, via the police.

The Health Act 2006 introduced the concept of an 'accountable officer' (see section 3.7.10) and requires healthcare organisations, and those providing services to healthcare organisations, to have standard operating procedures in place for using and managing Controlled Drugs.

For registered pharmacies, the Responsible Pharmacist Regulations 2008 also require that a range of pharmacy procedures are established – including procedures for controlled drugs (see Appendix 10).

3.7.2 CLASSIFICATION

The 2001 Regulations classify controlled drugs into five schedules according to the different levels of control attributed to each:

- Schedule 1 (CD Lic POM)
- Schedule 2 (CD POM)
- Schedule 3 (CD No Register POM)
- Schedule 4 (CD Benz POM and CD Anab POM)
- Schedule 5 (CD INV P and CD INV POM)

Information regarding the CD schedule of medicines with monographs is available within the British National Formulary for schedule 1 to schedule 4 medicines. A database for the classification of medicines including controlled drugs is available from the Royal Pharmaceutical Society website.

Schedule 1 (CD Lic POM)

Most schedule 1 drugs have no therapeutic use and a licence is generally required for their production, possession or supply. Examples include hallucinogenic drugs (e.g. 'LSD'), ecstasy-type substances, raw opium and cannabis. Sativex is a cannabinoid extract schedule 1 drug that does have a therapeutic use and has been exempted by the Home Office from licensing requirements. See section 3 for practical guidance on dealing with prescriptions for Sativex.

Schedule 2 (CD POM)

Pharmacists and other classes of person named in the 2001 Regulations have a general authority to possess, supply and procure schedule 2 controlled drugs when acting in that capacity.

Schedule 2 includes opiates (e.g. diamorphine, morphine, methadone), major stimulants (e.g. amphetamines) and quinalbarbitone.

Schedule 3 (CD No Register POM)

Schedule 3 controlled drugs include minor stimulants and other drugs (such as buprenorphine, temazepam, midazolam and phenobarbital) that are less likely to be misused (and less harmful if misused) than those in schedule 2.

Schedule 4 (CD Benz POM or CD Anab POM)

Schedule 4 is split into two parts:

- Part I (CD Benz POM) – contains most of the benzodiazepines and ketamine
- Part II (CD Anab POM) – contains most of the anabolic and androgenic steroids, together with clenbuterol (an adrenoceptor stimulant) and growth hormones

Schedule 5 (CD Inv POM or CD Inv P)

Schedule 5 contains preparations of certain controlled drugs (such as codeine, pholcodine and morphine) that are exempt from full control when present in medicinal products of specifically low strengths.

Table 8 summarises the various characteristics of controlled drugs.

TABLE 8: SUMMARY OF VARIOUS CHARACTERISTICS OF CONTROLLED DRUGS

	SCHEDULE 2	SCHEDULE 3	SCHEDULE 4 (PART 1)	SCHEDULE 4 (PART II)	SCHEDULE 5
DESIGNATION	CD POM	CD No Reg POM	CD Benz POM	CD Anab POM	CD Inv P or CD Inv POM
PRESCRIPTION REQUIREMENTS – SEE SECTION 3.7.7	Yes	Yes, except temazepam	No	No	No
PRESCRIPTION VALID FOR	28 days	28 days	28 days	28 days	6 months
ADDRESS OF PRESCRIBER REQUIRED TO BE WITHIN THE UK	Yes	Yes	No	No	No
PRESCRIPTION IS REPEATABLE*	No	No	Yes	Yes	Yes
REQUISITION NECESSARY	Yes	Yes	No	No	No
REQUISITION TO BE MARKED BY THE SUPPLIER	Yes	Yes	No	No	No
INVOICES TO BE RETAINED FOR TWO YEARS	No	Yes	No	No	Yes
LICENCE REQUIRED TO IMPORT OR EXPORT	Yes	Yes	Yes	Yes *(unless the substance is in the form of a medicine and for self-administration)*	No

* By 'repeatable' we mean the instance where the prescriber adds an instruction on the main prescription for the prescribed item to be repeated e.g. repeat x 3. This does not refer to the prescription counterpart which is sometimes used as a patient repeat request to the prescriber. NHS prescriptions are not repeatable.

3.7.3 POSSESSION AND SUPPLY

Pharmacists, doctors and dentists, when acting in these capacities, are among those empowered by the 2001 Regulations under a general authority to possess, supply and procure schedule 2, 3, 4 and 5 controlled drugs.

Other mechanisms for the lawful possession of controlled drugs include:

- **HOME OFFICE LICENCE** – persons who have an applicable Home Office licence can possess and supply controlled drugs in accordance with the terms of the licence (e.g. the museum of the Royal Pharmaceutical Society holds a Home Office licence to possess controlled drugs for the purposes of the museum)

- **HOME OFFICE GROUP AUTHORITY** – persons who are covered by an applicable Home Office licence group authority can possess and supply controlled drugs in accordance with the terms of the group authority (e.g. there is currently a group authority covering paramedics that allows them to possess and supply certain controlled drugs)

- **LEGISLATION: CLASS OF PERSON** – other classes of person specified in the 2001 Regulations, provided they are acting in the capacity of the specified class (e.g. a postal operator or, for specified controlled drugs, a registered practising midwife)

- **LEGISLATION: CLASS OF DRUG** – the 2001 Regulations indicate that possessing certain classes of controlled drugs is lawful (e.g. schedule 4 part II drugs when contained in medicinal products and schedule 5 drugs)

- **PATIENTS** – persons who have been prescribed a controlled drug by a doctor, supplementary prescriber, nurse independent prescriber, pharmacist independent prescriber, dentist or veterinary surgeon (for an animal)

A comprehensive analysis of the multiple classes of persons who and organisations that can possess and supply controlled drugs is outside the scope of this document. However, this has been summarised within Chapter 17 of Dale and Appelbe's *Pharmacy Law and Ethics* (London: Pharmaceutical Press; 2009) or can be found in the 2001 Regulations.

Possession of schedule 1 controlled drugs

A Home Office licence would be required to possess schedule 1 controlled drugs (with the exception of Sativex). However some pharmacists, particularly those working within a hospital, may be asked to deal with substances removed from patients on admission, which may be schedule 1 products (e.g. cannabis). A pharmacist, under two specific exemptions, can take possession of such controlled drugs. The first exemption is when possession is taken for the purpose of destruction. The second is for the purpose of handing over to a police officer.

The patient's confidentiality should normally be maintained and the police should be called on the understanding that the source will not be identified. If, however, the quantity is so large that the drug could not be purely for personal use the pharmacist may decide that the greater interests of the public require identification of the source. Such a decision should not be taken without first considering discussing the situation with the other health professionals involved in the patient's care and taking advice from the pharmacist's professional indemnity insurer's legal adviser.

The patient should give authority for the drug to be removed and destroyed. If the patient refuses, the pharmacist may feel that he or she has no alternative other than to call in the police. Under no circumstances can a suspected illicit drug be handed back to a patient.

3.7.4 ADMINISTRATION

Schedule 1 controlled drugs may only be administered, or prescribed under a Home Office licence. Sativex is a schedule 1 controlled drug which benefits from a Home Office licence and is discussed further in section 3.7.13.

Schedule 2, 3 or 4 controlled drugs can be administered to a patient by:

- A doctor, dentist, pharmacist independent prescriber or nurse independent prescriber acting in their own right

- A supplementary prescriber (including a pharmacist supplementary prescriber) acting in accordance with a clinical management plan

- A person acting in accordance with the directions of a prescriber entitled to prescribe controlled drugs (including pharmacist independent prescribers)

Since 23 April 2012, pharmacist independent prescribers have been empowered to be able to prescribe schedule 2, 3, 4 and 5 controlled drugs, administer them in their own right or direct their administration.

Only medical prescribers who hold a special licence from the Home Secretary can prescribe cocaine, diamorphine or dipipanone for treating addiction. This special licence is not required if treating organic disease or injury. Pharmacist independent prescribers, nurse independent prescribers and supplementary prescribers may not prescribe cocaine, diamorphine or dipipanone for treating addiction, but may prescribe these medicines for treating organic disease or injury.

NB: In healthcare environments, including secure environments additional requirements and restrictions regarding who may administer or witness the administration of medicines may exist to satisfy medicines management, governance and patient safety considerations.

3.7.5 IMPORT, EXPORT AND TRAVELLERS

A licence is needed for a pharmacy to import or export schedule 1, 2 or 3 controlled drugs. There are no restrictions on the import or export of schedule 4 part II medicines or schedule 5 controlled drugs (see Table 8).

Pharmacists are often asked about arrangements for patients who are taking controlled drugs abroad. The Home Office is the regulatory body in this instance and may require individuals to apply for personal licences in certain circumstances. Information can be found on the Home Office website (**www.homeoffice.gov.uk**).

TRAVELLERS

At the time of writing, a personal licence was not required by the Home Office if a person travelling is carrying less than three months' supply of a controlled drug. However, it is advised that a covering letter from the prescriber is obtained that confirms the name of the patient, travel plans, name of the prescribed controlled drug, total quantities and dose.

The patient should also check with the embassies or high commissions for the countries they will be travelling through to ensure that the import and export regulations in those countries are complied with.

It would be prudent for patients to check any additional requirements that their travel operator may impose.

3.7.6 OBTAINING CONTROLLED DRUGS – REQUISITION REQUIREMENTS FOR SCHEDULE 1, 2 AND 3 CONTROLLED DRUGS

Following the Shipman Inquiry, standardised controlled drug requisition forms have been introduced as a matter of good practice and specific forms are available for England, Scotland and Wales (see Table 9).

It is lawful for a supply to be made against a non-standard requisition form provided all the legal requirements are included. However, the Royal Pharmaceutical Society strongly recommends that the standard form is used routinely wherever possible. In a prison, hospital-style requisition forms (instead of a standardised form) are usually used and are printed in a bound, book format – sequentially numbered with a carbon copy of each requisition to provide a robust audit trail.

THE LEGAL REQUIREMENTS FOR A CONTROLLED DRUG REQUISITION ARE:

1. Signature of the recipient
2. Name of the recipient
3. Address of the recipient
4. Profession or occupation
5. Total quantity of drug
6. Purpose of the requisition

PRACTICE ISSUES

- Supplies made against a faxed or photocopied requisition are not acceptable

- Legislation requires that a requisition in writing must be obtained by the supplier before delivery of any schedule 2 or 3 controlled drug to most recipients – including practitioners, hospitals, care homes, ship and offshore installation personnel, supplementary prescribers, senior registered nurses in charge of wards, theatres and other hospital departments. Some recipients (such as other registered pharmacies) are not included in this legal requirement. However, for audit purposes, and as a matter of best practice, we would advise that supplies should only be made after receiving a written requisition. Therefore, where one registered pharmacy supplies another

registered pharmacy, as a matter of good practice, a requisition written on a standardised form should be obtained

- In an emergency, a doctor or dentist can be supplied with a schedule 2 or 3 controlled drug on the undertaking that a requisition will be supplied within the next 24 hours. Failure to do so would be an offence on the part of the doctor or dentist

- Where stock is collected by a messenger on behalf of a purchaser, a written authorisation must be provided to the supplying pharmacist that empowers the messenger to receive the medicines on behalf of the purchaser. The supplying pharmacist needs to be reasonably satisfied that the authorisation is genuine and must retain it for two years

TABLE 9: STANDARDISED REQUISITION FORMS

	ENGLAND	SCOTLAND	WALES
FORM THAT SHOULD BE USED	FP10CDF	CDRF – for private supplies GP10A – for NHS supplies	WP10CDF
WHERE TO OBTAIN FORMS	Local primary care trust	Local NHS health board	Local NHS health board

PROCESSING REQUISITION FORMS (MARKING AND SENDING)

When a valid requisition for a schedule 1, 2 or 3 controlled drug is received, it is a legal requirement to:

- Mark the requisition indelibly with the supplier's name and address (i.e. the name of the pharmacy) – where a pharmacy stamp is used this must be clear and legible

- Retain a copy of the requisition for two years from the date of supply

- Send the original requisition to the relevant NHS agency

These requirements are exempted when the supply is made:

- By a hospital or care homes (retain the original requisition for two years)

- By pharmaceutical manufactures or wholesalers

- By a prison pharmacy to wings within the prison

- Against a midwife supply order (see below)

- Against veterinary requisitions (the original requisition should be retained for five years)

Midwife supply orders

A registered midwife may use a midwife supply order to obtain the following controlled drugs:

- Diamorphine
- Morphine
- Pethidine

The order must contain the following:

- Name of the midwife
- Occupation of the midwife
- Purpose for which the controlled drug is required
- Total quantity of the drug to be obtained
- Signature of an appropriate medical officer – a doctor authorised (in writing) by the local supervising authority or the person appointed by the supervising authority to exercise supervision over midwives within the area

UNDERPINNING KNOWLEDGE

3.7.7 PRESCRIPTION REQUIREMENTS FOR SCHEDULE 2 AND 3 CONTROLLED DRUGS

The requirements that must be present for a prescription for schedule 2 or 3 controlled drugs to be valid are outlined in Diagram 6.

Pharmacy Stamp	Age	Title, Forename, Surname & Address:
		9 PATIENT NAME
	D.o.B.	**10** PATIENT ADDRESS

Please don't stamp over age box

Number of days' treatment
NB Ensure dose is stated | NHS Number:

Endorsements

4 DOSE

5 FORMULATION

6 STRENGTH

7 TOTAL QUANTITY

8 QUANTITY PRESCRIBED

11 DENTAL WORDING WHERE APPROPRIATE

12 INSTALMENT WORDING WHERE APPROPRIATE

EXAMPLE

Signature of Prescriber | Date

1 SIGNATURE OF PRESCRIBER | **2** DATE

For dispenser No. of Prescns. on form

3 ADDRESS OF PRESCRIBER

NHS

DIAGRAM 6: CONTROLLED DRUG PRESCRIPTION REQUIREMENTS FOR SCHEDULE 2 OR 3 CONTROLLED DRUGS

1 SIGNATURE – the prescription needs to be signed by the prescriber with their usual signature. The pharmacist should either recognise the signature (and believe it to be genuine) or take reasonable steps to satisfy themselves that it is genuine. The prescription may be signed by another prescriber other than the named prescriber and still be legally valid. However, the address of the prescriber needs to be applicable to the signatory for the prescription to be legally compliant. The controlled drugs register entry should record the details of the actual prescriber (the signatory) rather than the named prescriber. Doctors, dentists, vets, supplementary nurse or pharmacist prescribers (subject to a clinical management plan), independent nurse prescribers and pharmacist independent prescribers can prescribe controlled drugs. Advanced electronic signatures cannot be accepted for schedule 2 or 3 controlled drugs

2 DATE – the prescription needs to include the date on which it was signed. Controlled drugs prescriptions are valid for 28 days after the appropriate date on the prescription. The appropriate date is either the signature date or any other date indicated on the prescription (by the prescriber) as a date before which the drugs should not be supplied – whichever is later. The 28 day restriction applies to prescriptions for temazepam, schedule 4 controlled drugs and any owing balances

3 **PRESCRIBER'S ADDRESS** – the address of the prescriber must be included on the prescription and must be within the UK

4 **DOSE** – the dose does not need to be in both words and figures however it must be clearly defined (see Table 10)

5 **FORMULATION** – the formulation must be stated; the abbreviations "tabs" and "caps" are acceptable

6 **STRENGTH** – the strength only needs to be written on the prescription if the medicine is available in more than one strength. To avoid ambiguity, where a prescription requests multiple strengths of a medicine, each strength should be prescribed separately (i.e. separate dose, total quantity, etc)

7 **TOTAL QUANTITY** – the total quantity must be written in both words and figures. If the medicine is in dosage units (tablets, capsules, ampoules, millilitres, etc), the Home Office advises this must be expressed as a number of dosage units (e.g. 10 tablets [of 10mg] rather than 100mg total quantity). The total quantity can be expressed as the multiplication of two numbers provided both components are clearly and unambiguously written in words and figures (e.g. "2 packs of 30 tablets; two packs of thirty tablets"). Liquids should be expressed as millilitres

8 **QUANTITY PRESCRIBED** – the Department of Health and the Scottish Government have issued strong recommendations that the maximum quantity of schedule 2, 3 or 4 controlled drugs prescribed should not exceed 30 days. This is not a legal restriction but prescribers should be able to justify the quantity requested (on a clinical basis) if more than 30 days' supply is prescribed. There may be genuine circumstances for which medicines need to be prescribed in this way

9 **NAME OF PATIENT**

10 **ADDRESS OF PATIENT** – if the patient does not have a fixed address (e.g. because he or she is homeless or under a witness protection scheme), "no fixed abode" or "NFA" is acceptable. Use of a PO Box is not acceptable

11 **DENTAL PRESCRIPTIONS** – where the controlled drug prescription is written by a dentist, the words "for dental treatment only" should be present

12 **INSTALMENT DIRECTION** – where the prescription is intended to be supplied in instalments a valid instalment direction is required (see below)

Additional requirements: When the controlled drug is supplied, it is a requirement to mark the prescription with the date of supply. The prescription needs to be written in indelible ink and can be computer generated

Name of the medicine

Clearly, the name of the prescribed medicine is necessary on a prescription to identify which medicine is being requested. However, it is not a legal requirement. It is good practice to write the name of the medicine in full as it appears in the manufacturer's summary of product characteristics.

TABLE 10: EXAMPLES OF DOSES THAT ARE, AND ARE NOT, LEGALLY ACCEPTABLE

EXAMPLES OF DOSES THAT ARE NOT LEGALLY ACCEPTABLE	EXAMPLES OF DOSES THAT ARE LEGALLY ACCEPTABLE (NB: LEGAL ACCEPTABILITY DOES NOT AUTOMATICALLY INDICATE CLINICAL APPROPRIATENESS)
As directed	One as directed
When required	Two when required
PRN	One PRN
As per chart	Three ampoules to be given as directed
Titration dose	(better still – three ampoules to be given
Weekly (this is just a frequency and not a dose)	over 24 hours as directed)
Decrease dose by 3.5ml every four days	

Temazepam is a schedule 3 controlled drug that is exempt from usual schedule 2 and 3 controlled drug prescription form requirements. The supply restriction of 28 days after the appropriate date still applies (see Date). An advanced electronic signature cannot be accepted.

Instalment direction for schedule 2 or 3 controlled drugs

An instalment direction combines two pieces of information:

1. Amount of medicine per instalment
2. Interval between each time the medicine can be supplied

The Home Office has confirmed that an instalment prescription must have both a dose and an instalment amount specified separately on the prescription.

The first instalment must be dispensed within 28 days of the appropriate date (see Date). The remainder of the instalments should be dispensed in accordance with the instructions (even if this runs beyond 28 days after the appropriate date).

If the only date on the prescription is the date of signing, the first dispensing needs to take place within 28 days of this date. If the prescriber indicates on the prescription a date before which the prescribed medicine should not be dispensed, this would be the appropriate date instead. The prescription must then be marked with the date of each supply.

The instalment direction is a legal requirement and needs to be complied with. However, because there are acknowledged practical difficulties with missed doses and dates when the pharmacy is closed (e.g. bank holidays), the Home Office has approved specific wording to be used that gives pharmacists a degree of flexibility when making a supply.

The following wording allows a pharmacy to supply the balance of an instalment if the interval date is missed (i.e. if three days' supply was directed to be supplied on day 1 but it was missed, it allows two days' supply to be issued on day 2).

APPROVED WORDING FOR MISSED DOSE – SUPERVISED CONSUMPTION

"Supervised consumption of daily dose on specified days; the remainder of supply to take home. If an instalment prescription covers more than one day and is not collected on the specified day, the total amount prescribed less the amount prescribed for the day(s) missed may be supplied."

APPROVED WORDING FOR MISSED DOSE – UNSUPERVISED CONSUMPTION

"Instalment prescriptions covering more than one day should be collected on the specified day; if this collection is missed the remainder of the instalment (i.e. the instalment less the amount prescribed for the day[s] missed) may be supplied."

OR "If an instalment prescription covers more than one day and is not collected on the specified day, the total amount prescribed less the amount prescribed for the days missed may be supplied."

APPROVED WORDING IF THE PRESCRIBER WISHES TO ENSURE THAT THE PATIENT IS NOT SUPPLIED WITH ANY DOSES –

PROVIDED NO MORE THAN THREE DAYS HAVE BEEN MISSED

"Instalment prescriptions covering more than one day should be collected on the specified day. If this collection is missed, the remainder of the instalment (i.e. the total amount less the instalments for the days missed) may continue to be supplied in the specified instalments at the stated intervals, provided no more than three days are missed."

APPROVED WORDING FOR WHEN THE PHARMACY IS CLOSED

"Instalments due on days when the pharmacy is closed should be dispensed on the day immediately prior to closure."

NB: If the prescriber selects instalment intervals that take bank holidays or other closure dates into account, it may not be necessary to include this wording.

NB: If you decide to supply against a prescription that uses wording not approved by the Home Office, it will not provide the same protection from enforcement when making the supply. In this instance, if practical, you should try to get the prescription amended by the prescriber to include the approved Home Office wording.

Missed doses

If you know a patient has missed three days' prescribed treatment (or the number of days defined by any local agreement with the prescriber), there is a risk that he or she will have lost tolerance to the drug and the usual dose may cause overdose. In the best interests of the patient, consider contacting the prescriber to discuss appropriate next steps.

Technical errors

Where a prescription for a schedule 2 or 3 controlled drug contains a minor typographical error or spelling mistake, or where either the words or figures (but not both) of the total quantity has been omitted, a pharmacist can amend the prescription indelibly so that it becomes compliant with legislation.

The pharmacist needs to have exercised due diligence, be satisfied that the prescription is genuine and that the supply is in accordance with the intention of the prescriber. The prescription should also be marked to show that the amendments are attributable to the pharmacist (e.g. name, date, signature and GPhC registration number).

Pharmacists cannot correct other amendments or omissions (e.g. missing date, incorrect dose, form or strength). These should be corrected by the original prescriber or, in an emergency, another prescriber authorised to prescribe controlled drugs. Amendments cannot be made by covering letter from the prescriber.

> Only medical prescribers who hold a special licence from the Home Secretary can prescribe cocaine, diamorphine or dipipanone for treating addiction. This special licence is not required if treating organic disease or injury. Pharmacist independent prescribers, nurse independent prescribers and supplementary prescribers may not prescribe cocaine, diamorphine or dipipanone for treating addiction, but may prescribe these medicines for treating organic disease or injury.

Private prescription requirements for schedule 2 and 3 controlled drugs

I. STANDARDISED FORM

Following from the recommendations of the Shipman Inquiry, private prescriptions for schedule 2 or 3 controlled drugs (including temazepam) must be written on designated standardised forms. The forms that should be used are:

- FP10PCD – in England
- PPCD(1) – in Scotland
- WP10PCD – in Wales

Private prescriptions that are not on the designated standardised form must not be accepted unless they are veterinary prescriptions.

For a hospital pharmacy to lawfully supply a schedule 2 or 3 controlled drug against a private prescription issued outside that hospital (i.e. outside its legal entity),

a standardised form must be used. Where the private prescription is issued and dispensed within the same legal entity, a standardised form is not required.

2. PRESCRIBER IDENTIFICATION NUMBER

A prescriber identification number must be included on standardised private prescriptions. This number is not the prescriber's professional registration number (i.e. the GMC number). It is a number issued by the relevant NHS agency and can be obtained from the local primary care organisation. In Scotland, a valid NHS prescriber code is used where available or new ones issued where necessary.

3. SUBMISSION

Pharmacies must submit the original private prescription to the relevant NHS agency (NHS Business Services Authority or equivalent). This requires an identifying code assigned to the pharmacy for this purpose by the local primary care organisation.

Veterinary prescriptions for controlled drugs do not need to be written on standardised forms nor do they need to be submitted to the relevant NHS agency. Forms must be retained for five years.

The Veterinary Pharmacists Group virtual network is available to members on the RPS website (**www.rpharms.com**).

3.7.8 COLLECTION OF DISPENSED CONTROLLED DRUGS

When a schedule 2 controlled drug is collected from a pharmacy, the pharmacist is legally required to determine whether the person collecting is a patient, patient's representative or healthcare professional. Depending upon which type of person is collecting, the pharmacist needs to take appropriate action (see Table 11).

TABLE 11: ACTIONS REQUIRED WHEN A DISPENSED CONTROLLED DRUG IS COLLECTED

PERSON COLLECTING	ACTION	NOTES
PATIENT	Unless already known to the pharmacist, request evidence of identity	The decision whether to supply or not is at the discretion of the supplying pharmacist – based on their professional judgment
PATIENT'S REPRESENTATIVE		
HEALTHCARE PROFESSIONAL ACTING IN THEIR PROFESSIONAL CAPACITY ON BEHALF OF THE PATIENT	Unless already known to the pharmacist, obtain: 1. Name of healthcare professional 2. Address of healthcare professional Also request evidence of identity	Where evidence of identity is not available, the pharmacist has discretion over whether to supply or not – based on their professional judgment

Collection by a representative of a drug misuse patient

If a drug misuser wants a representative to collect a dispensed controlled drug on his or her behalf, pharmacists are advised to first obtain a letter from the drug misuser that authorises and names the representative. (This includes those detained in police custody who should supply a letter of authorisation to a police custody officer to present to the pharmacist). A separate letter must be obtained each time the drug misuser sends a representative to collect and the representative should bring identification. The pharmacist must be satisfied that

the letter is genuine. It is also good practice to insist on seeing the patient in person at least once a week unless this is known not to be possible.

If the directions on the prescription state that the dose must be supervised, the pharmacist should contact the prescriber before the medicine is supplied to the representative – since supervision will not be possible. It is legally acceptable to confirm verbally with the prescriber that they are happy with this arrangement since supervision, while important, is not a legal requirement under the 2001 Regulations. An appropriate record of this conversation should be made.

PRACTICE ISSUES

- It is good practice for the person collecting a schedule 2 or 3 controlled drug to sign the space on the reverse of the prescription form that is specifically for this purpose. A supply can be made if this is not signed, subject to the professional judgment of the pharmacist

- Instalment prescriptions only need to be signed once

- A representative, including a delivery driver, can sign on behalf of a patient. However, a robust audit trail should be available to confirm successful delivery of the medicine to the patient

3.7.9 SAFE CUSTODY

The concept of safe custody is derived from the Safe Custody Regulations and refers to the physical security of certain schedule 2 or 3 controlled drugs. It requires that pharmacies, private hospitals and care homes keep relevant controlled drugs in a "locked safe, cabinet or room which is constructed as to prevent unauthorised access to the drugs". For settings other than those listed above, these regulations are considered minimum standards for safe custody.

Structural requirements of safes, cabinets and rooms used for storing controlled drugs

The structural requirements and technical details with which controlled drug safes, cabinets and rooms must comply are detailed in schedule 2 of the Safe Custody Regulations. These requirements are of a technical nature requiring expertise and knowledge of construction. The Royal Pharmaceutical Society does not endorse or approve individual (or brands of) controlled drugs cabinets.

When purchasing a safe or cabinet, reassurance should be sought from the vendor or manufacturer that the product specifications comply with the requirements specified in the Safe Custody Regulations.

Alternatively, you must apply for an exemption certificate from the police, which certifies that the safe, cabinet or room provides an adequate degree of security for holding controlled drugs. For further information, contact your local police station.

The controlled drugs that must be kept under safe custody are:

- Schedule 1 drugs except Sativex (which should be stored in a lockable fridge or in a fridge in a secure location away from public view)

SAFE CUSTODY REQUIREMENTS FOR SECURE ENVIRONMENTS AND SECONDARY CARE

Prison building regulations specify details of the robust nature required for all rooms that store controlled drugs. For further information, see the Ministry of Justice's PSI 45/2010 Prison Service Order for Integrated Drug Treatment System (**www.nta.nhs.uk/uploads/psi_2010_45_idts.pdf**).

In prisons and hospitals, it is recommended that the CD cabinet should meet the "Sold Secure silver standard". For further information, see:

- **National Prescribing Centre.** *A guide to good practice in the management of controlled drugs in primary care* (England). December 2009. (**www.npc.nhs.uk**)

- **Department of Health.** *Safer management of controlled drugs: A guide to good practice in secondary care* (England). October 2007. (**www.dh.gov.uk**)

- Technical specifications for general design of storage facilities for healthcare facilities are available from the Space for Health website. (**www.spaceforhealth.nhs.uk**)

- Schedule 2 drugs except some liquid preparations and quinalbarbitone (secobarbital). Details of exempted schedule 2 controlled drugs are available from the Misuse of Drugs (Safe Custody) Regulations 1973 as amended

- Schedule 3 drugs unless exempted under the Misuse of Drugs (Safe Custody) Regulations 1973 as amended where the full lists are available. Common exemptions include: phenobarbital, mazindol, meprobamate, midazolam, pentazocine and phentermine

- Common schedule 3 controlled drugs which require safe custody include temazepam and buprenorphine

You may wish to keep other controlled drugs (i.e. those exempted from requiring safe custody) in the controlled drugs safe, cabinet or room if there is enough space. This can act as a reminder that these drugs are controlled drugs so may have other requirements (e.g. prescription requirements, etc).

When controlled drugs requiring safe custody are not kept in the controlled drugs cabinet, safe or room (e.g. during the dispensing process), they must be under the "direct personal supervision" of a pharmacist.

Access to controlled drugs (including handling of "CD keys") should be documented within a policy. The policy should prevent unauthorised access and be able to identify who has had access to controlled drugs (e.g. the electronic logs from a room or cabinet with electronic access or an audit trail for holders of the CD keys). In community pharmacies, it is common for the pharmacist to hold the CD keys.

Patient returned and out-of-date or obsolete controlled drugs

Safe custody applies to patient returned, out-of-date and obsolete controlled drugs until they can be destroyed (see section 3.7.10). To minimise the risk of supplying these to patients, this stock must be segregated from other pharmacy stock and be clearly marked (e.g. mark the stock as "patient returns waiting to be destroyed" or "out of date, waiting authorised witness to destroy", etc).

Pharmacies are required to denature controlled drugs prior to disposal. Usually, this process requires an appropriate licence but pharmacies are exempt from needing one (although they must register their exemption). Registration of an exemption is different from obtaining a licence.

In England and Wales, an exemption is issued by the Environment Agency and is known as the "T28 exemption". This allows pharmacies to sort and dispose of controlled drugs and to comply with the 2001 Regulations by denaturing them prior to disposal. This exemption needs to be registered with the Environment Agency, which can be done on their website (**www.environment-agency.gov.uk**).

In Scotland, the exemption is issued by the Scottish Environment Protection Agency (SEPA), which currently accepts that the denaturing of controlled drugs forms part of the exempt activity of secure storage.

Both the Environment Agency and SEPA have indicated that they may reconsider their positions at any time and may pursue enforcement action where activities cause, or are likely to cause, environmental pollution or harm to human health.

Controlled drugs that need to be denatured before disposal

The Home Office has advised that all controlled drugs in schedules 2, 3 and 4 (part 1) should be denatured and, therefore, rendered irretrievable before disposal.

Persons authorised to witness the denaturing of controlled drugs

In some circumstances, the denaturing of controlled drugs needs to be witnessed by an authorised person. Where there is a requirement to make a controlled drug register entry, legislation also requires to have their destruction witnessed. Typically, the destruction of pharmacy stock of schedule 2 controlled drugs needs to be witnessed. The destruction of patient returned controlled drugs, whether they require denaturing or not, does not require witnessing.

Table 12 summarises the denaturing and witnessing requirements for patient-returned and expired controlled drugs.

TABLE 12: DENATURING AND WITNESS REQUIREMENTS FOR PATIENT-RETURNED AND EXPIRED CONTROLLED DRUGS

	IS DENATURING REQUIRED?	IS AN AUTHORISED WITNESS REQUIRED?	RECORD KEEPING
PATIENT-RETURNED CONTROLLED DRUG	Yes, if schedule 2, 3 or 4 (part 1)	No. However it is preferable for denaturing to be witnessed by another member of staff familiar with controlled drugs.	A record should not be made in the controlled drugs register but records of patient returned schedule 2 controlled drugs and their subsequent destruction should be recorded in a separate record for this purpose.
EXPIRED STOCK	Yes, if schedule 2, 3 or 4 (part 1)	Yes, if schedule 2. For schedule 3 medicines it would be good practice to have another member of staff witness the denaturing.	An entry should be made in the controlled drug register for schedule 2 controlled drugs.

NB: If a pharmacy is engaged in manufacturing, compounding, importing or exporting schedule 3 or 4 controlled drugs then record keeping arrangements apply. Therefore, destruction of these requires an authorised witness.

In prisons, to maintain a robust audit trail, use of schedule 3 controlled drugs (e.g. buprenorphine) should be recorded in the controlled drugs register. Therefore, any destruction should also be recorded. It is also recommended that a robust audit trail is maintained for schedule 4 controlled drugs, such as diazepam and chlordiazepoxide.

Various individuals and classes of person (e.g. police constables) are authorised to witness the destruction of controlled drugs. This authority is derived from the Home Secretary. It can also be derived from the Secretary of State for Health or from an accountable officer (see below).

Accountable officers

Following the Shipman Inquiry, accountable officers were introduced with responsibility for supervising and managing the use of controlled drugs in their organisation or setting. One of the many roles of accountable officers is to appoint authorised witnesses for the destruction of controlled drugs. Sources of information on the duties of accountable officers are specified in Table 13.

TABLE 13: SOURCES OF INFORMATION ON THE DUTIES OF ACCOUNTABLE OFFICERS AND LISTS OF ACCOUNTABLE OFFICERS

ENGLAND	The National Prescribing Centre has published a document that describes the core role of accountable officers. The resource is entitled the *Handbook of controlled drug accountable officers in England (1st edition)* and is available on the centre's website (**www.npc.nhs.uk**) A register of accountable officers in England is published on the Care Quality Commission website (**www.cqc.org.uk**)
SCOTLAND	Information on the role of accountable officers in Scotland is available in a Scottish Government Health Department letter (**www.sehd.scot.nhs.uk/mels/HDL2007_12.pdf**) A list of accountable officers in Scotland is available on the Scottish Government Head Directory website (**www.sehd.scot.nhs.uk**)
WALES	Information regarding the role of accountable officers in Wales and a list of accountable officers is available on the Healthcare Inspectorate Wales website (**www.hiw.org.uk**)

NB: An accountable officer has the power to authorise other persons to witness the destruction of controlled drugs. However the 2001 Regulations prevent an accountable officer from being an authorised person directly. Persons authorised by the accountable officer are usually senior members of staff who are not involved in the day-to-day management or use of controlled drugs.

Methods of denaturing controlled drugs

All medicines should be disposed of in a safe and appropriate manner. Medicines should be disposed of in appropriate waste containers that are then sent for incineration. They should not be disposed of into the sewerage system.

Table 14 specifies how controlled drugs should be destroyed – according to their type of formulation.

TABLE 14: DESTRUCTION OF CONTROLLED DRUGS

DOSAGE FORM	METHOD OF DESTRUCTION
TABLETS AND CAPSULES	Remove from outer packaging and, wearing gloves, remove from blister packaging and place into a CD denaturing kit (a commercial product designed to render controlled drugs irretrievable). Best practice would be to grind* or crush* the solid dosage formulation before adding to the CD denaturing kit to ensure that whole tablets or capsules are irretrievable An alternative method of denaturing is to crush or grind the solid dose formulation and place it into a small amount of hot, soapy water – stirring sufficiently to ensure the drug has been dissolved or dispersed. The resulting mixture, once cool, can then be added to an empty waste disposal container supplied by the waste contractor
LIQUID DOSE FORMULATIONS	Pour from container into a CD denaturing kit, which should then be placed into a pharmaceutical waste container Alternatively, pour onto an appropriate amount of cat litter (or similar product), taking into account Health and Safety Regulations so that the person destroying the drug and the environment are safeguarded from harm and pollution The cat litter (or similar product) should be disposed of by incineration via the usual waste disposal methods for medicines
AMPOULES	Wearing suitable protective gloves, ampoules containing liquid should be opened and the contents emptied into a CD denaturing kit or disposed of in the same manner as the disposal of liquid dose formulations above. The ampoule can then be disposed of in the sharps bin Wearing suitable protective gloves, ampoules containing powder can be opened and then have water added to dissolve the powder inside. The resulting mixture can then be poured into the CD denaturing kit. The ampoule can be disposed of in the sharps bin An alternative, but less preferable, disposal method is to crush the ampoules with a pestle inside an empty plastic container. Once broken, a small quantity of hot, soapy water (for powder ampoules) or cat litter (for liquid ampoules) is added. If these methods are used, care should be taken to ensure that the glass does not harm the person destroying the drug. The resulting liquid mixture should then be disposed of in a CD denaturing kit or in the bin that is used to dispose of liquid medicines
FENTANYL OR BUPRENORPHINE PATCHES	The active ingredient in the patches can be rendered irretrievable by removing the backing and folding the patch over on itself and then placing it in a waste disposal bin or, preferably, a CD denaturing kit. Gloves must be worn by the person destroying the patch
AEROSOL FORMULATIONS	Aerosol formulations should be expelled into water (to prevent droplets of drug entering the air). As a further precaution, a facemask should be worn by staff undertaking the activity. Also, it should be carried out in well ventilated area. The resulting solution can then be disposed of in accordance with the above guidance on destroying liquid formulations

*If grinding or crushing of tablets or capsules takes place, steps must be taken to ensure that particles of drug dust are not released into the air – or that this is minimised. The use of a small amount of water while grinding or crushing may assist. It may also be necessary for the person involved in the grinding or crushing to wear a suitable face mask for protection, suitable gloves and ensure that the area is well ventilated.

A controlled drugs register must be used to record details of any schedule 1 (except Sativex) and schedule 2 controlled drugs received or supplied by a pharmacy.

For controlled drugs **received**, the following must be recorded:

- Date supply received
- Name and address from whom received
- Quantity received

For controlled drugs **supplied**, the following must be recorded:

- Date supplied
- Name and address of recipient

- Details of authority to possess – prescriber or licence holder's details
- Quantity supplied
- Details of person collecting schedule 2 controlled drug – patient, patient's representative or healthcare representative (if the latter, also record their name and address)
- Whether proof of identity was requested of the person collecting
- Whether proof of identity was provided

These are the minimum fields of information that must be recorded; additional relevant information can be added without breaking the law.

THE NATURE OF THE REGISTER

Legislation requires that the class, strength and form be specified at the head of each page of the controlled drugs register. It is also a requirement that different classes are kept in a separate register or separate part of the register and that, within each class, a separate page is used for different strengths and formulations of each drug. Multiple registers for the same class of controlled drug are allowable if approved by the Home Office.

Prisons have one legally compliant register that records all the details as specified. However, since there are often several areas in each prison where controlled drugs are stored, administered or issued, each of these areas should maintain a controlled drug record book (similar to those used by hospital wards). Also recommended is that the movement of controlled drugs between these areas be recorded by internal requisition so that robust audit trails are maintained.

THE NATURE OF THE ENTRIES

All entries made in controlled drugs registers should be:

- **Entered chronologically**

- **Entered promptly** – entries must be made on the day of the transaction or on the following day
- **In ink or indelible** – entries and corrections must be in ink or indelible (or computerised [see below])
- **Unaltered** – entries must not be cancelled, obliterated or altered. Corrections must be made by dated marginal notes or footnotes

RECORD KEEPING

The following points regarding record keeping should be adhered to when maintaining controlled drugs registers:

- **Location** – each register should be kept at the premises to which it applies
- **Duration** – registers should be kept for two years from the date of the last entry
- **Form** – records can be kept in their original form or copied and kept in an approved computerised form
- **Inspection** – a copy of the register, and other details of stock, receipts and supplies, must be made available to authorised persons (e.g. a General Pharmaceutical Council inspector or controlled drug liaison officer) upon request

Running balances

The aim of a running balance is to ensure that irregularities or discrepancies are identified as quickly as possible. Balances should be checked with the physical amount of stock at regular intervals. This is normally weekly but may be more frequent if the volume of controlled drugs dispensed is high; if there are several different pharmacists in charge over short periods; or where there has been a past irregularity. With the exception of oral liquid dosage forms, it would also be appropriate to visually check the running balance each time a controlled drug is dispensed.

A running balance should be maintained as a matter of good practice and is a recommendation from the Shipman Inquiry. It is intended that once electronic registers are in common use this will become a legal requirement.

PRACTICE ISSUES

■ The pharmacist has overall responsibility for maintaining running balances and dealing with discrepancies. However these tasks can be delegated to competent staff, where appropriate

■ If a discrepancy can be resolved following checks, a marginal note or footnote should be made in the register and the discrepancy corrected

■ An SOP should be written for how to check running balances and deal with discrepancies. This SOP should include instructions for when the owner or superintendent, GPhC inspector, accountable officer or controlled drug liaison officer should be notified of discrepancies

■ Running balances for liquid controlled drugs can be affected by overage, residue and spillage

■ Where a CD register entry has been made for a schedule 2 controlled drug, the usual requirement to make a record in the POM register does not apply

ELECTRONIC CONTROLLED DRUGS REGISTERS

Electronic controlled drugs registers are permitted as an alternative to having a bound-book controlled drugs register. Legislation requires that computerised entries must be:

■ Attributable

■ Capable of being audited

■ Compliant with best practice

An electronic controlled drugs register must also be accessible from the premises and capable of being printed.

Registers may only be kept in computerised form if safeguards are incorporated into the software to ensure all of the following:

■ The author of each entry is identifiable

■ Entries cannot be altered at a later date

■ A log of all data entered is kept and can be recalled for audit purposes

Access control systems should be in place to minimise the risk of unauthorised or unnecessary access to the data. Adequate backups must be made of computerised registers. Arrangements should be made so that inspectors can examine computerised registers during a visit with minimum disruption to the dispensing process.

UNDERPINNING KNOWLEDGE

3.7.12 PRACTICE ISSUES: DISPOSING OF SPENT METHADONE BOTTLES

Legislation does not state how empty methadone bottles should be disposed. However the Department of Health has produced guidance about empty medicine containers. For liquid controlled drug containers, these should first be emptied as far as possible (within the dispensing process) and any excess liquid (e.g. patient returns) denatured. The container should then be placed into a waste container for incineration.

> **FURTHER READING**
>
> **Department of Health.** *Safe management of healthcare waste (version 1).* March 2011. (**www.dh.gov.uk**)

3.7.13 PRACTICE ISSUES: DISPENSING SCHEDULE 1 SATIVEX SPRAY

On 16 June 2010, Sativex, an oromucosal spray containing cannabidiol and delta-9-tetrahydrocannabinol in a 1:1 ratio, became available as a licensed product. Sativex, which is derived from whole plant extracts of the plant Cannabis sativa, is currently a schedule 1 controlled drug so pharmacists need to be aware of the legal and professional requirements and exemptions relating to its supply.

Prescribing

Prescriptions for Sativex should be written in accordance with the same prescription requirements as for schedule 2 controlled drugs. Under the terms of the Home Office general open licence, Sativex can only be prescribed by a doctor, and non-medical prescribers may not prescribe it.

Any amendments necessary to enable the supply of the licensed product must be undertaken by the prescribing doctor.

Private prescriptions for Sativex must be written on standardised private prescription forms

Record keeping

Under its general open licence, Sativex is exempt from the controlled drug record keeping requirements. Although pharmacists are not legally required to keep a record of its acquisition or supply in the controlled drug register, they can make entries to maintain an audit trail.

Storage requirements

For storage purposes, if a lockable fridge is available pharmacists are required (by the Home Office) to store Sativex in it. In the absence of a lockable fridge, Sativex should be stored in a fridge in a secure location and away from public view.

Sativex should be stored upright in a fridge (between 2 and 8°C) prior to opening. Once opened, it can be stored upright at room temperature for a maximum of 42 days.

What preparations are available for supply?

Previously Sativex was only available as an unlicensed import from Canada in 4 x 5.5ml pack sizes. The packs licensed in the UK are 3 x 10ml packs. The two products are bioequivalent and identical to each other, and differ only in volume.

Pharmacists should consult the prescribing doctor if a prescription is received for the unlicensed form because a licensed version is the preferred product.

The prescription will need to be amended by the prescriber regarding the number of packs and volume (i.e. quantity to supply).

> **FURTHER READING**
>
> **RPS Support.** *Sativex – quick reference guide.* October 2011. (**www.rpharms.com**)

3.7.14 PRACTICE ISSUES: DISPENSING AND PREPARING EXTEMPORANEOUS METHADONE

In April 2011 the GPhC issued a call for evidence on methadone preparation, the result of which could impact upon the appropriateness of extemporaneous preparation.

Methadone should only be dispensed extemporaneously if the quantity needed for regular dispensing requirements is too great for licensed methadone to be stored practically – i.e. subject to safe custody. A licensed product is nearly always preferable to the same unlicensed product. This is because products with a marketing authorisation must comply with high standards of manufacturing practice.

The following are important considerations if you are preparing and dispensing extemporaneous methadone:

Standard operating procedure – a robust SOP for the preparation of extemporaneous methadone must be in place and adhered to

TRAINING – only trained and competent persons can be involved in preparing extemporaneous methadone

EQUIPMENT

TYPE – appropriate equipment should be used to measure and prepare extemporaneous methadone. According to National Measurement Office guidance, weighing instruments for pharmaceuticals must be "high accuracy class 2 devices". For measuring liquid volumes, dispensing measures must comply with British Standard 1922 or the equivalent European standard

MAINTENANCE – all equipment should be maintained and in good order

CLEANING – any equipment used must be properly cleaned after each batch is prepared so that no residue remains

MEASUREMENT OF INGREDIENTS – all quantities of ingredients (including excipients) used for extemporaneous preparation of methadone must be measured accurately with appropriate equipment without relying on quantities stated by manufacturers

VISUAL CHECKS – extemporaneously prepared methadone should be visually checked to ensure that the methadone powder has dissolved fully in the diluent

PREPARATION – follow the directions on the prescription and consult, where applicable, a formula from a suitable formulary, pharmacopoeia, compendium or the manufacturer's instructions

LABELLING THE STOCK BOTTLE – the product should be labelled with:

- name and strength of the product
- quantity
- any special handling or storage requirements (e.g. store in safe custody)
- the batch expiry date
- a batch reference number

It is also good practice to label with the formulation.

STOCK BOTTLES – once a stock bottle has been used, it must not be re-used. Instead, it should be disposed of into the pharmaceutical waste bin and a new bottle used next time

STORAGE (SAFE CUSTODY) – after preparation, the product must be stored subject to safe custody (which, in most pharmacies, will mean within a controlled drugs cabinet)

RECORD KEEPING – for each batch prepared, a record should be made (e.g. in the controlled drugs register) and retained for two years. This record should include:

- the formula
- the ingredients and quantities used
- the source, batch number and expiry date of the ingredients
- the batch number and expiry date of the extemporaneously prepared mixture
- the persons involved in preparing the product, including the identity of the pharmacist assuming overall responsibility

CONTROLLED DRUGS REGISTER – appropriate entries should be made in the controlled drugs register. There must be an entry in when methadone powder is received and another entry out when the powder is used to prepare extemporaneous methadone. There then needs to be a separate entry in for the methadone liquid prepared

RUNNING BALANCE – a running balance should be used for the methadone powder and for extemporaneously prepared methadone liquid

INFORMING THE PATIENT AND PRESCRIBER – both the prescriber and the patient should be informed that the product supplied does not have a marketing authorisation

INDEMNITY – the increased liability associated with preparing extemporaneous methadone must be covered by adequate indemnity insurance.

FURTHER RESOURCES

Online resources available on the National Measurement Office website (**www.nmo.bis.gov.uk**)

4. ROYAL PHARMACEUTICAL SOCIETY RESOURCES

The following resources are available from our website (**www.rpharms.com**):

Pharmacy Law and Ethics

- Controlled drugs (October 2010)
- Dispensing and Preparing Extemporaneous Methadone (September 2010)
- EEA Prescriptions (December 2010)
- Emergency Supply (February 2011)
- Independent Prescribing of controlled drugs (April 2012)
- Legal Classifications of Medicines database
- Medicines, Ethics and Practice: A Guide for pharmacists
- Professional Judgment (September 2010)
- Professional Support Bulletins
- Pseudoephedrine and Ephedrine (September 2010)
- Responsible Pharmacist Toolkit
- Safe Custody of controlled drugs (August 2011)
- Sativex (October 2010)
- Supply of Medicines to Podiatrists and their patients
- Veterinary Medicines (October 2010)

Reclassified Medicines

- Amorolfine Nail Lacquer (May 2006)
- Azithromycin (November 2008)
- Chloramphenicol Eye Drops (November 2011)
- Omeprazole (May 2011)
- Orlistat (July 2011)
- Sumatriptan (June 2006)
- Tamsulosin (March 2010)
- Tranexamic Acid P Medicine (January 2011)

Pharmacy Practice

- 8 Core Principles for Community Pharmacy whistle blowing policies and procedures (September 2011)
- Advertising Pharmacy Services and Medication (August 2011)
- Best Practice for ensuring the efficient supply and distribution of medicines to patients (February 2011)
- Cholesterol Testing (December 2010)
- Clinical Governance (September 2011)
- Cough and Cold products for children (February 2011)
- Dispensing Oral Isotretinoin and pregnancy prevention (March 2012)
- Emergency Contraception (Updated September 2011)
- Good Dispensing guidelines – England (August 2009)
- Handling of Medicines in Social Care (replaces Administration and control of medicines in care homes and children's services) (2007)
- Homeopathic and Herbal products (February 2010)
- Ibuprofen, Isopropyl Myristate topical P medicine (February 2012)
- Identification of Foreign Medicines
- Medicines Adherence : NICE implementation guidance for Pharmacists (February 2009)
- Medical Devices (January 2012)
- Medicines that Optometrists can order (April 2012)
- Monitoring Blood pressure (January 2011)
- Near Miss Error Log (October 2010)
- Patient Group Directions: A resource pack for pharmacists (July 2008)
- Protecting Children and Young People (September 2011)
- Protecting Vulnerable Adults (November 2011)
- Raising concerns, whistle blowing and speaking up safely in Pharmacy (September 2011)

- Safe and Secure handling of Medicines
  (Revised Duthie Report – RPS Website)
- Specials (May 2010)
- Standards for the design of hospital in-patient
  prescription charts (September 2011)
- Standards for hospital pharmacy services
- The Traditional Herbal medicine registration scheme
  (June 2011)
- Transfer of Care (July 2011)

Clinical Aspects of Pharmacy

- Bowel Cancer (February 2012)
- Bowel Screening (April 2010)
- Clinical Check (May 2011)
- Counselling patients on medicine (August 2011)
- Diagnostic testing and screening services (March 2009)
- Diabetes (March 2010 – RPS Website)
- Dispensing and Supply of Oral Chemotherapy
  and Systemic Anticancer Medicines in Primary Care
  (January 2011 – RPS Website)
- How to use the BNF (June 2011)
- Improving practice and reducing risk in the provision
  of parental nutrition for neonates and children
  (December 2011 – RPS Website)
- Lung Cancer (October 2010)
- Medication History (May 2011)
- Ovarian Cancer (February 2012)
- Supporting patients with Asthma (September 2011)
- Supporting Patients with Chronic Obstructing
  Pulmonary Disease (COPD) (September 2011)
- Supporting patients on Oral Anticoagulants
  (March 2012)

Public Health Issues

- Alcohol use disorders (June 2010)
- Mental health (April 2010)
- Mental health toolkit (2010)
- Obesity and Weight management (June 2010)
- Seasonal Influenza (December 2010 – RPS Website)
- Sexual Health (March 2010 – RPS Website)
- Smoking Cessation (April 2011)

Online Resources

- CPD Case studies, guidance, FAQs, examples
  and templates
- E-Alert and RPS support updates
- E-library (Royal Pharmaceutical Society electronic
  library for access to books and full-text
  journal databases)
- Essential websites for pharmacists – online database
- Map of evidence – online database
- Mentoring online resources
- Pharmacy research and evaluation resources
- Qualified persons: Joint professional body
  eligibility scheme and support material
- Return to practice – online resources

Professional Standards for Hospital Pharmacy Services

OPTIMISING PATIENT OUTCOMES FROM MEDICINES. FOR PHARMACY SERVICES IN ACUTE, MENTAL HEALTH, PRIVATE AND COMMUNITY SERVICE PROVIDERS

In 2011, the RPS began a programme of work to develop professional standards for hospital pharmacy services. These professional standards aim to ensure that patients receive a high quality pharmacy service, from admission through to discharge across multiple care pathways. We have identified 1- overarching standards that underpin the patient experience, and the safe, effective management of medicines within and across organisations. They will enable patients to experience a consistent quality of service within and across healthcare providers that helps protect them from incidents of avoidable harm and enables them to get the best outcomes from their medicines.

The professional standards have been developed by the professional and facilitated by the RPS, in close partnership with Association of Teaching Hospital Pharmacists (ATHP), the Guild of Healthcare Pharmacists (GHP) and our RPS partner groups; with extensive input from our pharmacy advisory group, representing a broad range of hospital pharmacy services in acute, private and community settings, across all three countries.

At the time of production of this edition of MEP, publication of the new professional standards is imminent, and will be available on our website once published.

Office details for the Royal Pharmaceutical Society are:

HEAD OFFICE

1 Lambeth High Street
London SE1 7JN
Tel: 0845 257 2570 or 0207 572 2737
Fax: 020 7735 7629
Email: support@rpharms.com

SCOTTISH OFFICE

Holyrood Park House
106 Holyrood Road
Edinburgh EH8 8AS
Tel: 0131 556 4386
Fax: 0131 558 8850
Email: scotinfo@rpharms.com

WELSH OFFICE

Unit 2, Ashtree Court
Woodsy Close
Cardiff Gate Business Park
Cardiff CF23 8RW
Tel: 029 2073 0310
Fax: 029 2073 0311
Email: wales@rpharms.com

Details of how the Royal Pharmaceutical Society is governed are available on our website (**http://www.rpharms.com/about-us/how-we-are-governed.asp**)

Details of the current national pharmacy board members are available on the links below:

http://www.rpharms.com/english-pharmacy-board/english-pharmacy-board-members.asp

http://www.rpharms.com/scottish-pharmacy-board/scottish-pharmacy-board-members.asp

http://www.rpharms.com/welsh-pharmacy-board/welsh-pharmacy-board-members.asp

5. EXCLUDED TOPICS AND SIGNPOSTING

For some of the topics which have become less relevant to day-to-day pharmacy practice, and are no longer core within the new MEP, the following sources of information may be useful.

TABLE 15: EXCLUDED TOPICS AND SIGNPOSTING

TOPIC	REASON FOR EXCLUSION	ALTERNATIVE RESOURCE
HUMAN A–Z LIST OF MEDICINES	Limited use in day-to-day practice as information is available by marketing authorisation on the packaging of the medicine. Lists are not exhaustive and information exists elsewhere.	**RPS website:** remains available to members via online database and PDF **BNF:** CD schedule information and partial classification for medicines within formulary **MHRA:** Rama XL resource. Commercial access to comprehensive MHRA sentinel database. Available under subscription **Other:** C&D price list, OTC directories, Summary of Product characteristics database (**www.medicines.org.uk**), Home Office list of controlled drugs (**homeoffice.gov.uk**)
LISTS DERIVED FROM MEDICINES LEGISLATION E.G. WHOLESALE LISTS CONDITIONS UNDER WHICH SMALLPOX VACCINE CAN BE ADMINISTERED	Reproduction of legislation and lists from legislation is not a core role of a professional body. Some lists are of little relevance to daily practice. Alternative sources of information are also available.	Consolidation and simplified medicines legislation is expected to be available by July 2012. This will be available on the government legislation website (**www.legislation.gov.uk**) and it is anticipated that an up-to-date version will be available on the MHRA website (**www.mhra.gov.uk**) The consolidated legislation is expected to be the Human Medicines Regulations 2012 Dale and Appelbe's Pharmacy Law and Ethics 9th Edition
POISONS LISTS	No longer relevant to day-to-day practice	Dale and Appelbe's Pharmacy Law and Ethics 9th Edition Poisons List Order 1982 (**www.legislation.gov.uk**)

TOPIC	REASON FOR EXCLUSION	ALTERNATIVE RESOURCE
CHIP OR COSSH REGULATIONS	Comprehensive alternative source of information available	Comprehensive information available from the Health and Safety Executive. **www.hse.gov.uk/chip** **www.hse.gov.uk/coshh**
DENATURED ALCOHOL	Comprehensive alternative source of information available	Detailed information available in HMRC Notice 473
HEALTHCARE PROFESSIONAL ACTING IN THEIR PROFESSIONAL CAPACITY ON BEHALF OF THE PATIENT	Reliable and robust alternative sources of information freely available	Veterinary Medicines Directorate product database. (**www.vmd.defra.gov.uk**) NOAH compendium database (**www.noah.co.uk**)

EXCLUDED TOPICS AND SIGNPOSTING

6. PARTNERSHIPS WITH SPECIALIST GROUPS

The Royal Pharmaceutical Society is committed to collaborating and co-operating with partners from across the profession to advance pharmacy. We work in partnership with a wide range of specialist groups, many of whom have established networks, to ensure their specialist expertise and knowledge influences and informs the work of the RPS. We work with our partnership groups to ensure a strong voice for the profession and professional support and development for pharmacists working in all areas of pharmacy.

The following table contains details of the partners of the Royal Pharmaceutical Society, some brief information about each group and website details.

TABLE 16: SPECIALIST PARTNERSHIP GROUPS

PARTNERSHIP GROUP	ABOUT OUR PARTNER	DETAILS
AMBULANCE PHARMACISTS NETWORK (APN)	The Ambulance Pharmacists Network meets four times a year and is an opportunity for pharmacists working for ambulance services across the UK to share good medicines management practice.	**www.rpharms.com/ sector-groups/ambulance- pharmacists-network.asp**
ASSOCIATION OF PHARMACY TECHNICIANS (APTUK)	The Association of Pharmacy Technicians UK is the professional leadership body for pharmacy technicians working in the UK. The APTUK aims to work on behalf of pharmacy technicians and in partnership with other pharmacy organisations to help deliver professional excellence.	**www.aptuk.org**
BRITISH PHARMACEUTICAL NUTRITION GROUP (BPNG)	**A network for pharmacists**, pharmacy technicians, **scientists** and other healthcare professions with a **specialism or interest** in any aspect of nutrition, in particular **parenteral or enteral nutrition**. The aim of the group is to promote and develop best standards within nutrition and to provide high quality education on the subject.	**www.bpng.co.uk**
BRITISH ONCOLOGY PHARMACY ASSOCIATION (BOPA)	BOPA is the British Oncology Pharmacy Association and was formed to "promote excellence in the pharmaceutical care of patients with cancer through education, communication, research and innovation by an alliance of hospital, community and academic pharmacists, pharmacy technicians, those in the pharmaceutical industry and other healthcare professionals".	**www.bopawebsite.org**

PARTNERSHIP GROUP	ABOUT OUR PARTNER	DETAILS
BRITISH SOCIETY FOR THE HISTORY OF PHARMACY (BSHP)	The British Society for the History of Pharmacy was formed in 1967 having originated from a committee of the Royal Pharmaceutical Society. It seeks to act as a focus for the development of all areas of the history of pharmacy, from the works of the ancient apothecary to today's ever changing role of the community, wholesale or industrial pharmacist.	www.bshp.org
COLLEGE OF MENTAL HEALTH PHARMACY (CMHP)	The College of Mental Health Pharmacy promotes its members as recognised experts in the optimal use of medicines in improving mental health and supports them by a process of ongoing accreditation and education.	www.rpharms.com/clinical-and-pharmacy-practice/college-of-mental-health-pharmacy.asp
FACULTY OF CANCER PHARMACISTS (FCP)	The Faculty is a distinct, autonomous, professional body. It provides professional support for pharmacists in the UK, from any professional background, who are interested and/or working in the specialist area of cancer pharmacy. Launched in January 2008 as a joint venture between the college and The British Oncology Pharmacy Association, it is run by a working board consisting of six people elected from the membership, and works to a formal constitution.	www.rpharms.com/clinical-and-pharmacy-practice/faculty-of-cancer-pharmacy.asp
HIV PHARMACISTS ASSOCIATION (HIVPA)	HIVPA is the UK HIV Pharmacy Association which was established in 1991 and has a long history of providing high quality education, support and networking for its members to improve professional and personal development. Its membership is open to all pharmacists and technicians working in or with an interest in HIV, infectious diseases and sexual health. HIVPA organises highly educational study days with on line live streaming and a two day national conference every year. HIVPA's aim is to promote excellence in the pharmaceutical care of patients living with HIV. HIVPA recognises and promotes advanced pharmacy practice and supports research and collaboration with other health care professionals. HIVPA works closely with national HIV charities, campaigns and with the British HIV Association and is represented on several sub committees e.g. national treatment guidelines and contributes to the national standard documents.	www.hivpa.org

PARTNERSHIPS WITH SPECIALIST GROUPS

PARTNERSHIP GROUP	ABOUT OUR PARTNER	DETAILS
INSTITUTE OF PHARMACY MANAGEMENT (IPM)	The Institute of Pharmacy Management promotes education, research and excellence in pharmacy management. Incorporated in 1964 under the Companies Act as a Limited Company (By Guarantee), the Institute is essentially an educational body which is non-profit making. The Institute embraces all branches of pharmacy: community, hospital, academia, the pharmaceutical industry and wholesale distribution 10% of its 300 members live in some 20 countries outside the United Kingdom. Membership details can be found on our website our website.	**www.ipmi.org.uk**
JOINT PHARMACEUTICAL ANALYSIS GROUP (JPAG)	Study of pharmaceutical analysis and quality control by holding scientific meetings and promoting lectures, practical demonstrations and discussions''. JPAG has close contact with the industrial, academic, NHS and regulatory and enforcement sectors, and serves as the primary UK focus for those with an interest in any aspect of pharmaceutical analysis and related facets of medicines control and registration.	**www.rpharms.com/science- -research-and-technology/ joint-pharmaceutical-analysis- group.asp**
NATIONAL ASSOCIATION OF WOMEN PHARMACISTS (NAWP)	The National Association of Women Pharmacists was formed in June 1905 and has the mission of enabling all women pharmacists to realise their full potential and raise their profile by being educationally, socially and politically active. Membership is open to all UK pharmacists and former pharmacists (e.g. retired or taking a career break) and all UK pharmacy graduates, regardless of age or gender.	**www.nawp.org.uk**
NATIONAL PHARMACY CLINICAL TRIALS ADVISORY GROUP (NPCTAG)	The *National Pharmacy Clinical Trials Advisory Group (NPCTAG)*, originally a subgroup of the National Pharmaceutical Quality Assurance Committee, was established in its current form in 2010. Membership of NPCTAG includes representatives from a range of hospital pharmacy disciplines and other relevant specialist groups, MHRA and the National Institute of Health Research. The group's objectives are to: ■ Provide advice to NHS pharmacy services to the National Institute of Health Research Clinical Research Networks Coordinating Centre ■ Support education & training of pharmacy staff ■ Provide a forum for communication with MHRA about clinical trial issues	**www.rpharms.com/clinical- and-pharmacy-practice/ national-pharmacy-clinical- trials-network.asp**

PARTNERSHIP GROUP	ABOUT OUR PARTNER	DETAILS
NEONATAL AND PAEDIATRIC PHARMACY GROUP (NPPG)	The Neonatal and Paediatric Pharmacists Group (NPPG) was formed in 1994, with an aim to improve the care of neonates, infants and children by advancing the personal development of pharmacists and technicians through the provision of quality pharmacy services in relation to practice, research and audit, education and training, communication and advice.	**www.nppg.scot.nhs.uk**
PALLIATIVE CARE PHARMACISTS NETWORK (PCPN)	Membership of the Network is open to pharmacists working in palliative care, which for many may only be part of their role. Pharmacists from the community, hospital and Primary Care Trust (PCT) sectors are all also welcome.	**www.pcpn.org.uk**
PRIMARY AND COMMUNITY CARE PHARMACY NETWORK (PCCPN)	The Primary and Community Care Pharmacy Network is a UK-wide group of pharmacists and technicians who provide advice and services to community health professionals, social care and voluntary organisations, local authorities, carers and patients. Their expertise includes understanding provision of community health services and the standards required to a wide range of settings and services including in-patient services, community nursing, school health, outreach teams, residential and day care and community clinics. They work on behalf of their members to support them with their day-to-day practice, to promote the highest standards of practice and to help influence national policy and strategies affecting those services for which their members are responsible.	**www.networks.nhs.uk/ nhs-networks/primary-and- community-care-pharmacy- network**
PRIMARY CARE PHARMACISTS ASSOCIATION (PCPA)	The Primary Care Pharmacists' Association (PCPA) was established in 1999 for the benefit of all pharmacists with an active interest in primary care pharmacy. The PCPA is now the largest and longest-standing independent organisation dedicated to supporting pharmacists working within primary care.	**www.pcpa.org.uk**
PHARMACY LAW AND ETHICS ASSOCIATION (PLEA)	The Pharmacy Law and Ethics Association (PLEA) is an independent group for pharmacists who are interested in law and ethics and lawyers or ethicists who are interested in pharmacy. PLEA was founded in 1997 by Professor Joy Wingfield who is the current chairman.	**www.plea.org.uk**

PARTNERSHIPS WITH SPECIALIST GROUPS

PARTNERSHIP GROUP	ABOUT OUR PARTNER	DETAILS
NHS PHARMACEUTICAL QUALITY ASSURANCE COMMITTEE	The NHS Quality Assurance Committee is made up of the lead Quality Assurance Specialists from the four home nations of the United Kingdom. The committee acts as a point of liaison between the NHS and the MHRA on matters affecting the manufacture of medicines in the NHS and regularly provides national guidance on many aspects of technical pharmacy service provision in NHS hospital pharmacy practice. Current chairman: Mark Jackson, Tel 0151 794 8110 mark.jackson@lrippu.nhs.uk	**www.qcnw.nhs.uk**
RADIOPHARMACISTS GROUP (UKRPG)	The origins of the UK Radiopharmacy Group date from 1976 and an initiative by a small group of practising radiopharmacists to work together for the advancement of radiopharmacy.	**www.bnms.org.uk/general/ ukrg-homepage.html**
SECURE ENVIRONMENT PHARMACISTS GROUP (SEPG)	The SEPG is a special interest group for pharmacists providing professional services to prisons and other secure environments in England and Wales. The group is open to all pharmacists directly providing services to or with organisational responsibility for, medicines management in these locations.	**www.rpharms.com/sector-groups/secure-environment-pharmacists-group.asp**
UNITED KINGDOM CLINICAL PHARMACY ASSOCIATION (UKCPA)	The UK Clinical Pharmacy Association (UKCPA) is a member association for clinical pharmacy practitioners. We encourage, support and promote advanced practice in pharmacy. The UKCPA actively develops clinical pharmacy practice as well as developing individual practitioners, and we are frequently at the forefront of initiatives such as establishing professional curricula, developing professional recognition (credentialing) processes, and developing professional tools and frameworks for practitioners. The Association was established in 1981 with the aim of bringing together like-minded pharmacists from different practice areas to share knowledge, research and experiences. This remains our core aim today. We provide networking and educational opportunities for our members to discuss and resolve current clinical issues and share best practice. In April 2011 the UKCPA became an official partner of the pharmacy professional body, the Royal Pharmaceutical Society and we work closely with other specialist pharmacy organisations, professional bodies and representatives of healthcare professions.	**www.ukcpa.org**

PARTNERSHIP GROUP	ABOUT OUR PARTNER	DETAILS
UNITED KINGDOM MEDICINES INFORMATION (UKMI)	UKMi is the United Kingdom Medicines Information network – a pharmacist-led service that helps patients and healthcare professionals working in all sectors to use medicines safely and effectively. We provide evidence-based, tailored advice on the pharmaceutical care of individual patients; we also produce a portfolio of innovative products designed to help clinicians, managers, and commissioners deliver high-quality cost-effective services. UKMi is a virtual network in which local patient-focussed services in acute-Trusts are advanced, developed, and supported regionally and nationally. There are around 220 local medicines information centres facilitated by 16 larger ones serving specific geographies; centres pool resource to work under the UKMi banner. National standards underpin the work of medicines information pharmacists and pharmacy technicians, who have both clinical expertise and particular skills in locating and interpreting information about medicines. Through UKMi, pharmacists and pharmacy technicians have access to various training resources and short courses, an active discussion forum, and both regional and national development and networking events.	**www.ukmi.nhs.uk**
UK OPHTHALMIC PHARMACY GROUP(UKOP)	The UK Ophthalmic Pharmacy Group aim to promote and develop ophthalmic care within pharmacy, particularly in the hospital setting. To develop members' knowledge of the ophthalmology specialty, and to discuss and share experiences in ophthalmic care.	**www.eyetext.net/opg**
UNITED KINGDOM RENAL PHARMACY GROUP (UKRPG)	The UK Renal Pharmacy Group (UKRPG) aims to promote excellence in the provision of pharmaceutical services to renal patients and associated healthcare professionals. To this end the Renal Pharmacy Group (UKRPG) publishes and encourages the dissemination of relevant information amongst pharmacists, pharmacy technicians, students and associated healthcare professionals, working in partnership with pharmacy colleagues from other specialties. The UKRPG also actively contributes to, and promotes, pharmaceutical research, audit and innovation in renal medicine and pharmacy practice.	**www.renalpharmacy.org.uk/ index.php**

7. PHARMACIST SUPPORT

Pharmacist Support (formerly the benevolent fund of the Royal Pharmaceutical Society) is an independent charity working for the welfare of pharmacists and their families, pre-registration trainees and pharmacy students in times of need. Services that this organisation provides include:

- Listening friends
- Specialist advice services
  (e.g. employment law, benefits and debt)
- Health support programme
- Grants and financial assistance

The general helpline for Pharmacist Support is 0808 168 2233 and further information can be found on its website (**www.pharmacistsupport.org**).

APPENDICES

Appendices 1 to 11 are standards, guidance and interim standards that have been reproduced with the kind permission of the General Pharmaceutical Council (GPhC). These documents are subject to change and review by the GPhC and the latest versions can be obtained from the GPhC website (**www.pharmacyregulation.org**).

The GPhC Standards Team can be contacted at:

Standards Team
General Pharmaceutical Council
129 Lambeth Road
London SE1 7BT

Phone: 0203 365 3460

Email: standards@pharmacyregulation.org

At the time of the production of MEP 36, the GPhC had consulted on new standards for registered pharmacies which are intended to replace their interim standards for pharmacy owners and superintendent pharmacists of retail pharmacy businesses. The new standards will be considered by the GPhC Council in September 2012.

APPENDIX 1:   GPhC STANDARDS OF CONDUCT, ETHICS AND PERFORMANCE

APPENDIX 2:   INTERIM GPhC STANDARDS FOR PHARMACY OWNERS AND
                SUPERINTENDENT PHARMACISTS OF RETAIL PHARMACY BUSINESSES

APPENDIX 3:   GPhC STANDARDS FOR CONTINUING PROFESSIONAL DEVELOPMENT

APPENDIX 4:   GPhC GUIDANCE ON PATIENT CONFIDENTIALITY

APPENDIX 5:   GPhC GUIDANCE ON CONSENT

APPENDIX 6:   GPhC GUIDANCE ON RAISING CONCERNS

APPENDIX 7:   GPhC GUIDANCE ON MAINTAINING CLEAR SEXUAL BOUNDARIES

APPENDIX 8:   GPhC GUIDANCE ON THE PROVISION OF PHARMACY SERVICES AFFECTED
                BY RELIGIOUS AND MORAL BELIEFS

APPENDIX 9:   GPhC GUIDANCE FOR OWNERS AND SUPERINTENDENT PHARMACISTS
                WHO EMPLOY RESPONSIBLE PHARMACISTS

APPENDIX 10:   GPhC GUIDANCE FOR RESPONSIBLE PHARMACISTS

APPENDIX 11:   GPhC GUIDANCE ON RESPONDING TO COMPLAINTS AND CONCERNS

APPENDIX 1: GPhC STANDARDS OF CONDUCT, ETHICS AND PERFORMANCE

This document sets out the standards of conduct, ethics and performance that pharmacy professionals must follow. Pharmacy professionals are pharmacists and pharmacy technicians who are registered with us. It is important that you meet our standards and that you are able to practise safely and effectively. Your conduct will be judged against the standards and failure to comply could put your registration at risk. If someone raises concerns about you we will consider these standards when deciding if we need to take any action. The work of a pharmacy professional can take many forms and you may work in different settings, including clinical practice, education, research and industry.

If you are a pharmacy professional these standards apply to you, even if you do not treat, care for or interact directly with patients and the public. As well as standards of conduct, ethics and performance, we publish other standards which you need to consider together with these standards. To help you to understand these standards, we have published a glossary of terms. We will also publish guidance to advise you on what you will need to do to meet these standards. The glossary and our guidance can be found on our website at **www.pharmacyregulation.org**.

The Seven Principles

As a pharmacy professional, you must:

1. Make patients your first concern
2. Use your professional judgment in the interests of patients and the public
3. Show respect for others
4. Encourage patients and the public to participate in decisions about their care
5. Develop your professional knowledge and competence
6. Be honest and trustworthy
7. Take responsibility for your working practices

We do not dictate how you should meet our standards. Each standard can normally be met in more than one way and the way in which you meet our standards may change over time. The standards are of equal importance. You are professionally accountable for your practice. This means that you are responsible for what you do or do not do, no matter what advice or direction your manager or another professional gives you. You must use your professional judgment when deciding on a course of action and you should use our standards as a basis when making those decisions. You may be faced with conflicting professional or legal responsibilities. In these circumstances you must consider all possible courses of action and the risks and benefits associated with each one to decide what is in the best interests of patients and the public.

1. MAKE PATIENTS YOUR FIRST CONCERN

The care, well-being and safety of patients are at the heart of professional practice. They must always be your first concern. Even if you do not have direct contact with patients your decisions or behaviour can still affect their care or safety.

YOU MUST:

1.1 Make sure the services you provide are safe and of acceptable quality

1.2 Take action to protect the well-being of patients and the public

1.3 Promote the health of patients and the public

1.4 Get all the information you require to assess a person's needs in order to give the appropriate treatment and care

1.5 If you need to, refer patients to other health or social care professionals, or to other relevant organisations

1.6 Do your best to provide medicines and other professional services safely and when patients need them

1.7 Be satisfied that patients or their carers know how to use their medicines

1.8 Keep full and accurate records of the professional services you provide in a clear and legible form

1.9 Make sure you have access to the facilities, equipment and resources you need to provide your professional services safely and effectively

1.10 Organise regular reviews, audits and risk assessments to protect patient and public safety and to improve your professional services

2. USE YOUR PROFESSIONAL JUDGMENT IN THE INTERESTS OF PATIENTS AND THE PUBLIC

Balancing the needs of individuals with those of society as a whole is essential to professional practice.

YOU MUST:

2.1 Consider and act in the best interests of individual patients and the public

2.2 Make sure that your professional judgment is not affected by personal or organisational interests, incentives, targets or similar measures

2.3 Make the best use of the resources available to you

2.4 Be prepared to challenge the judgment of your colleagues and other professionals if you have reason to believe that their decisions could affect the safety or care of others

2.5 In an emergency, consider all available options and do your best to provide care and reduce risks to patients and the public

3. SHOW RESPECT FOR OTHERS

Showing respect for other people is essential in forming and maintaining professional relationships.

YOU MUST:

3.1 Recognise diversity and respect people's cultural differences and their right to hold their personal values and beliefs

3.2 Treat people politely and considerately

3.3 Not unfairly discriminate against people. Make sure your views about a person's lifestyle, religion or belief, race, gender reassignment, identity, sex and sexual orientation, age, disability, marital status or any other factors, do not affect how you provide your professional services

3.4 Make sure that if your religious or moral beliefs prevent you from providing a service, you tell the relevant people or authorities and refer patients and the public to other providers

3.5 Respect and protect people's dignity and privacy. Take all reasonable steps to prevent accidental disclosure or unauthorised access to confidential information. Never disclose confidential information without consent unless required to do so by the law or in exceptional circumstances

3.6 Get consent for the professional services you provide and the patient information you use

3.7 Use information you obtain in the course of your professional practice only for the purposes you were given it, or where the law says you can

3.8 Make sure you provide the appropriate levels of privacy for patient consultations

3.9 Maintain proper professional boundaries in your relationships with patients and others that you come into contact with during the course of your professional practice and take special care when dealing with vulnerable people

4. ENCOURAGE PATIENTS AND THE PUBLIC TO PARTICIPATE IN DECISIONS ABOUT THEIR CARE

Patients and the public have a right to be involved in decisions about their treatment and care. This needs effective communication. You should encourage patients and the public to work in partnership with you and others to manage their needs.

YOU MUST:

4.1 Communicate effectively with patients and the public and take reasonable steps to meet their communication needs

4.2 Work in partnership with patients and the public, their carers and other professionals to manage their treatment and care. Listen to patients and the public and respect their choices

4.3 Explain the options available to patients and the public, including the risks and benefits, to help them make informed decisions. Make sure the information you give is impartial, relevant and up to date

4.4 Respect a person's right to refuse to receive a professional service

4.5 Make sure that information is appropriately shared with other health and social care professionals involved in the care of the patient

4.6 Consider and take steps, when possible, to address those factors that may be preventing or deterring patients from getting or taking their treatment

4.7 If a person cannot legally make decisions about their care, make sure that any service you provide is in line with the appropriate legal requirements

5. DEVELOP YOUR PROFESSIONAL KNOWLEDGE AND COMPETENCE

Up-to-date and relevant professional knowledge and skills are essential for safe and effective practice. You must ensure that your knowledge, skills and performance are of a high standard, up to date and relevant to your field of practice at all stages of your professional working life.

YOU MUST:

5.1 Recognise the limits of your professional competence. Practise only in those areas in which you are competent to do so and refer to others if you need to

5.2 Maintain and improve the quality of your practice by keeping your knowledge and skills up to date and relevant to your role and responsibilities

5.3 Apply your knowledge and skills appropriately to your practice

5.4 Learn from assessments, appraisals and reviews of your professional performance and undertake further education and training if necessary

5.5 Undertake and keep up-to-date evidence of your continuing professional development.

6. BE HONEST AND TRUSTWORTHY

Patients and the public put their trust in pharmacy professionals. You must behave in a way that justifies this trust and maintains the reputation of your profession.

YOU MUST:

6.1 Act with honesty and integrity to maintain public trust and confidence in your profession

6.2 Not abuse your professional position or exploit the vulnerability or lack of knowledge of others

6.3 Avoid conflicts of interest and declare any personal or professional interests you have. Do not ask for or accept gifts, rewards or hospitality that may affect, or be seen to affect, your professional judgment

6.4 Be accurate and impartial when you teach and when you provide or publish information. Do not mislead or make claims that you have no evidence for or cannot justify

6.5 Meet accepted standards of personal and professional conduct

6.6 Comply with legal and professional requirements and accepted guidance on professional practice

6.7 Keep to your commitments, agreements and arrangements to provide professional services

6.8 Respond honestly, openly and politely to complaints and criticism

6.9 Promptly tell us, your employer and all relevant authorities about anything that may mean you are not fit to practise or that may damage the reputation of the pharmacy professions. This includes ill health that affects your ability to practise, criminal convictions and findings of other regulatory bodies or organisations.

7. TAKE RESPONSIBILITY FOR YOUR WORKING PRACTICES

Working in a team is an important part of professional practice and relies on respect, co-operation and communication between colleagues from your own and other professions. When you work as part of a team you are accountable for your own decisions and behaviour and any work you supervise.

YOU MUST:

7.1 Practise only if you are fit to do so

7.2 Make sure that you and everyone you are responsible for have the language skills to communicate and work effectively with colleagues

7.3 Contribute to the development, education and training of colleagues and students, and share your knowledge, skills and expertise

7.4 Take responsibility for all work you do or are responsible for. Make sure that you delegate tasks only to people who are trained to do them, or who are being trained

7.5 Make sure it is clear who is responsible for providing a particular service when you are working in a team

7.6 Be satisfied that appropriate standard operating procedures are in place and are being followed

7.7 Make sure that you keep to your legal and professional responsibilities and that your workload or working conditions do not present a risk to patient care or public safety

7.8 Make sure that your actions do not stop others from keeping to their legal and professional responsibilities, or present a risk to patient care or public safety

7.9 Make sure that all your work, or work that you are responsible for, is covered by appropriate professional indemnity cover

7.10 Make sure that there is an effective complaints procedure where you work and follow it at all times

7.11 Make the relevant authority aware of any policies, systems, working conditions, or the actions, professional performance or health of others if they may affect patient care or public safety. If something goes wrong or if someone reports a concern to you, make sure that you deal with it appropriately

7.12 Co-operate with any investigations into your or another healthcare professional's fitness to practise and keep to undertakings you give or any restrictions placed on your practice because of an investigation

APPENDIX 2: INTERIM GPhC STANDARDS FOR PHARMACY OWNERS AND SUPERINTENDENT PHARMACISTS OF RETAIL PHARMACY BUSINESSES

This document sets out the standards for pharmacy owners and superintendent pharmacists in relation to carrying on a retail pharmacy business at a registered pharmacy premises. These terms are defined in our glossary. We have set these standards to protect patients and the public and to promote the safe and effective practice of pharmacy at registered pharmacies. If you are responsible for providing pharmacy services within your organisation you must make sure that all the standards set out in this document are met, whether you do that directly or delegate that responsibility to someone else. This includes where you delegate your responsibilities to a non-pharmacist manager.

This document does not detail legislative requirements, but when in a position of authority you must comply with the legislative and contractual requirements, such as NHS terms of service, relevant to your management responsibilities. You must also meet our standards of conduct, ethics and performance which are published in a separate document. To help you to understand these standards, we have published a glossary of terms. We will also publish guidance to advise you on what you will need to do to meet these standards.

1. MANAGEMENT AND LEADERSHIP RESPONSIBILITIES

Owners and superintendent pharmacists have overall responsibility for setting out the standards and policies for the provision of pharmacy services by their organisations. Where a body corporate owns a pharmacy business, a superintendent pharmacist must be appointed to manage the pharmaceutical aspects of the business. Superintendent pharmacists have legal obligations under the Medicines Act 1968. The role of superintendent pharmacist is a key position carrying full-time responsibility and accountability within a company. If you are undertaking these roles, your professional obligations are explained below.

AS A MEMBER OF A BOARD OF A BODY CORPORATE YOU MUST:

1.1 Consider and act on the advice of the superintendent pharmacist when dealing with the requirements of the pharmaceutical parts of the business

1.2 Provide the superintendent pharmacist with the necessary support and resources to carry out their legal and professional obligations

1.3 Notify us in writing of any changes of superintendent pharmacist or to the address or ownership of a registered pharmacy premises

AS AN OWNER OR A SUPERINTENDENT PHARMACIST YOU MUST:

1.4 Identify and manage risks to patients, the public and those you employ

1.5 Set the overarching standards and policies for the pharmaceutical aspects of the business

1.6 Manage the keeping, preparing, dispensing and sale or supply of medicinal products and medical devices by a registered retail pharmacy business

1.7 Ensure that all legal and professional requirements are adhered to

1.8 Respond appropriately to any systems failures or concerns that may arise

1.9 Make sure that the responsible pharmacist is supported to fulfil their legal and professional responsibilities and appropriate systems are in place to deal with concerns raised by the responsible pharmacist

1.10 Make sure clear lines of accountability exist and that a retrievable audit trail of the health professional taking responsibility for the provision of each pharmacy service is maintained

1.11 Be satisfied that there are appropriate policies setting out the number of staff and their required experience and that they are made known to relevant staff

1.12 Make sure all professional activities undertaken by you or under your control are covered by adequate professional indemnity cover

1.13 Declare to the relevant person or authority any interests that could be perceived to influence your judgment in financial or commercial dealings which impact on patient care or public safety

1.14 Be satisfied that any advertising and promotional activity for professional services or medicines is legal, decent and truthful and complies with appropriate advertising codes of practice

1.15 Make sure products that may be injurious to a person's health, for example tobacco products, alcoholic beverages and products intended to mask the signs of alcohol or drug consumption, are not sold or supplied from registered pharmacy premises

AS A SUPERINTENDENT PHARMACIST YOU MUST:

1.16 Be satisfied that you have sufficient resources, authority and influence within your organisation to comply with your legal and professional responsibilities

1.17 Make sure that the members of the board of the body corporate are aware of and understand your responsibilities

1.18 Retain overall professional accountability for the pharmaceutical aspects of the business even if you are employed for fewer hours than the pharmacy business operates

2. POLICIES, PROCEDURES AND RECORDS

For the safe and effective running of a pharmacy it is essential that appropriate policies, procedures and records are established, maintained and reviewed. You must ensure that all legal and professional requirements are met in relation to the pharmacy services.

YOU MUST:

RECORD-KEEPING MECHANISMS

2.1 Make sure records are accurate, up to date and accessible

2.2 Make sure records are clear and legible

2.3 Keep records secure and confidential

STANDARD OPERATING PROCEDURES

2.4 Make sure there are standard operating procedures for all aspects of the safe and effective provision of pharmacy services, and these are maintained and regularly reviewed

2.5 Be satisfied that procedures respect and protect confidential information about patients and employees in accordance with current legislation, relevant codes of practice and professional guidelines

INCIDENT-REPORTING MECHANISMS

2.6 Have a method of recording incidents that is accessible and available

2.7 Regularly review incidents recorded and take appropriate action where necessary to ensure that risks to patients, the public and others are minimised

HANDLING COMPLAINTS AND MANAGING CONCERNS

2.8 Make sure there is an appropriate mechanism to respond to and investigate all complaints and concerns from patients and the public, pharmacy staff and others

2.9 Be satisfied that patients and the public, pharmacy staff and others know how to complain and raise concerns

2.10 Keep appropriate records of any complaints or concerns and action taken

3. PHARMACY STAFF

Employees must be supported when carrying out their professional and legal duties. They must be provided with training and development opportunities to strengthen and improve their knowledge, skills and competencies. You must make sure that staff are employed, managed and trained appropriately.

YOU MUST:

EMPLOYING, MANAGING OR LEADING OTHERS

3.1 Make sure your staff have or will undertake appropriate training to attain the skills, knowledge and competency, including sufficient language competence for their role

3.2 Be satisfied that staff understand their individual roles and responsibilities, including the activities and decisions which have and have not been delegated to them

3.3 Be satisfied that staff have appropriate supervision, either directly or through a managed system with clear reporting structures

3.4 Be satisfied that staff are able to comply with their professional and legal responsibilities

3.5 Be satisfied that staff are able to exercise their professional judgment in the best interest of patients and the public

3.6 Carry out appropriate checks before employment commences

3.7 Make sure staff are able to take appropriate rest breaks and encourage them to do so

TRAINING STAFF

3.8 Give staff access to the training they need and make sure they undertake any accredited training requirements relevant to their duties in a timely manner

3.9 Regularly review the progress and performance of staff, particularly trainees, and give honest and constructive feedback.

3.10 When training pre-registration trainee pharmacists and pharmacy technicians be satisfied:

- the trainee is fit to practise throughout their training contract

- the training meets the development needs of the trainee and provides the necessary range of experiences of professional practice

- the trainee is appropriately supervised and monitored by their pre-registration tutor or supervisor and their performance is honestly and impartially evaluated

- pre-registration training is provided in approved premises and we are notified when such training is being provided

4. PHARMACY PREMISES

The pharmacy premises from which services are provided must be safe and fit for purpose. You must ensure that the premises you own or are the superintendent for are appropriate for the professional services being provided.

YOU MUST:

THE CONDITIONS OF THE PREMISES

4.1 Be satisfied that the pharmacy premises you are responsible for are safe and fit for purpose and do not bring the pharmacy profession into disrepute

4.2 Clearly identify the premises from which professional services are provided and make sure they are well maintained

THE AVAILABILITY OF FACILITIES AND EQUIPMENT AT THE PREMISES

4.3 Make sure the facilities and equipment necessary to provide professional services are available in the pharmacy

4.4 Be satisfied the facilities and equipment are of an appropriate quality for the safe and effective provision of services

THE CONDITIONS IN WHICH MEDICINAL PRODUCTS ARE TO BE STORED

4.5 Store medicines, pharmaceutical ingredients, devices and other stock at the pharmacy premises or other locations under suitable conditions that take into account the stability of the drug

ARRANGEMENTS FOR THE OBTAINING, HANDLING, USE, SUPPLY AND SECURITY OF MEDICINAL PRODUCTS OR MEDICAL DEVICES

4.6 Make sure systems are in place to ensure that the supplier and the quality of any medicines, devices and pharmaceutical ingredients obtained are reputable

4.7 Put in place procedures so that medicines or medical devices that are out-of-date, returned from patients, obsolete or otherwise not suitable for supply are not supplied, except in exceptional circumstances or where medical devices are designed or intended for re-use

4.8 Ensure medicines and medical devices are disposed of safely

4.9 Ensure medicines, pharmaceutical ingredients, devices and other stock are kept securely

4.10 Ensure systems are in place for the safe supply of medicines to patients and the public

4.11 Ensure products with a marketing authorisation
are supplied where such products exist in a
suitable form and are available, in preference to
unlicensed products or food supplements except
where an exemption has been authorised (the
GPhC has authorised an exemption to enable
the extemporaneous preparation of methadone)

4.12 Ensure procedures for sales of over the counter
medicines enable intervention and professional advice
to be given whenever this can assist the safe and
effective use of medicines. Pharmacy medicines must
not be accessible to the public by self-selection.

4.13 Ensure systems are in place to manage and report
suspected counterfeit medicines

OPERATING AN INTERNET PHARMACY SERVICE

4.14 Have systems in place to protect and maintain
data integrity

4.15 Be satisfied that patients and the public who use
your internet service are readily able to identify:

- the name of the owner of the business

- the address of the registered pharmacy
premises at which the business is conducted

- where applicable, the name of the superintendent
pharmacist

- information about how to confirm the registration
status of the pharmacy and pharmacist

- details of how to make a complaint about the
on-line services provided

APPENDIX 3: GPhC STANDARDS FOR CONTINUING PROFESSIONAL DEVELOPMENT

This document sets out the standards for continuing professional development (CPD). It is important that you meet our standards and that you are able to practise safely and effectively. The CPD requirements apply equally to all pharmacy professionals. They are not changed by factors such as part-time employment, or working in a position of authority. You are expected to cover the full scope of your practice in your CPD record, including responsibilities such as superintendent or pharmacist prescriber and roles in different settings such as industry and community pharmacy. Your conduct will be judged against the standards and failure to comply could put your registration at risk.

If someone raises concerns about you we will consider these standards when deciding if we need to take any action. To help you to understand these standards, we have published a glossary of terms. We will also publish guidance to advise you on what you will need to do to meet these standards. The glossary and our guidance can be found on our website at **www.pharmacyregulation.org**.

Patients, the public and government expect that every pharmacy professional maintains their professional capability throughout their career. Keeping a record of your CPD enables you to confirm that you are meeting these expectations. It also helps you to retain and build your confidence as a professional and it will provide evidence that you meet our CPD requirement.

1.1 Keep a record of your CPD that is legible, either electronically online at the website **www.uptodate.org.uk**, on another computer, or as hard copy on paper and in a format published or approved by us and carrying the CPD approved logo

1.2 Make a minimum of nine CPD entries per year which reflect the context and scope of your practice as a pharmacist or pharmacy technician

1.3 Keep a record of your CPD that complies with the good practice criteria for CPD recording published in Plan and Record by us (**www.pharmacyregulation.org**)

1.4 Record how your CPD has contributed to the quality or development of your practice using our CPD framework

1.5 Submit your CPD record to us on request

APPENDIX 4: GPhC GUIDANCE ON PATIENT CONFIDENTIALITY

This guidance should be read alongside the **standards of conduct, ethics and performance** which all pharmacists and pharmacy technicians must apply to their practice. This document gives guidance on standards 3.5, 3.7 and 3.8 of the standards of conduct, ethics and performance, which say:

- You must respect and protect people's dignity and privacy. Take all reasonable steps to prevent accidental disclosure or unauthorised access to confidential information. Never disclose confidential information without consent unless required to do so by the law or in exceptional circumstances.

- You must use information you obtain in the course of your professional practice only for the purposes you were given it, or where the law says you can.

- You must make sure you provide the appropriate levels of privacy for patient consultations.

This document gives guidance to pharmacy professionals on how to meet the standards on confidentiality. The guidance is not intended to cover every issue and it does not give detailed legal advice. However, it reflects the current law in Great Britain.

You should use your professional judgment in applying this guidance in your own practice. You must make sure that you keep up to date and comply with the law, for example: the Data Protection Act 1998, the Human Rights Act 1998, and the common law duty of confidentiality, and with any NHS or employment policies on confidentiality that apply to your particular area of work.

You must make sure that all staff members you are responsible for are aware of this guidance and appropriately trained in all areas that are relevant to their duties. If you are not sure about what you should do in a specific situation, you should always ask for advice from your employer, your professional indemnity insurance provider, your professional body or other pharmacy organisation, or get independent legal advice.

We have produced more guidance to help pharmacy professionals apply our standards of conduct, ethics and performance. You can find this on our website. In particular, when reading this guidance you should also see our 'Guidance on consent'.

1 DUTY OF CONFIDENTIALITY

1.1 You have a professional and legal duty to keep confidential the information you obtain during the course of your professional practice. Maintaining confidentiality is a vital part of the relationship between a pharmacy professional and a patient. Patients may be reluctant to ask for advice, or give you the information you need to provide proper care, if they believe that you may not keep the information confidential. Your duty of confidentiality applies to everyone whatever their age (See our guidance on consent).

1.2 The duty of confidentiality applies to all information you obtain during the course of your professional practice.

1.3 Confidential information includes:

- electronic and hard copy data

- personal details

- information about a person's medication (prescribed and non-prescribed)

- other information about a person's medical history, treatment or care that could identify them, and

- information that patients or the public share with you that is not strictly medical in nature.

1.4 Confidential information does not include:

- anonymous information – information from which individuals cannot reasonably be identified

- coded information – information from which individuals cannot reasonably be identified, but which enables information about different patients to be distinguished (for example to identify drug side effects)

- information that is already legitimately in the public domain.

2 PROTECTING INFORMATION

2.1 It is essential that you take steps to protect the confidential information you are given in the course of your professional practice. You must:

- take all reasonable steps to protect the confidentiality of information you receive, store, send or destroy

- store hard copy and electronic documents, records, registers, prescriptions and other sources of confidential information securely. Do not leave confidential information where it may be seen or accessed by patients, the public or anyone else who should not have access to it

- take steps to prevent accidental disclosure of confidential information

- not discuss information that can identify patients where the discussions can be overheard by others not involved in their care

- not disclose information on any websites, internet chat forums or social media that could identify a patient

- make sure that everyone who works in your pharmacy knows about their responsibility to maintain confidentiality

- raise concerns with the person with responsibility for data control where you work, or with any other appropriate authority, if you find that the security of personal information on the premises where you work is not appropriate

- continue to protect a person's confidentiality after they have died, subject to disclosures required by law or when it is in the public interest (see below).

3 DISCLOSING CONFIDENTIAL INFORMATION

3.1 Decisions about disclosing confidential information can be complex. In most situations you do not have to disclose information immediately. However, there will be limited situations where to delay is not practical, for example if this may cause risk to another person. You should take the necessary steps to satisfy yourself that any disclosure sought is appropriate and meets the legal requirements covering confidentiality.

3.2 Maintaining confidentiality is an important duty, but there are circumstances when it may be appropriate to disclose confidential patient information. These are:

- when you have the patient's consent, or
- when the law says you must, or
- when it is in the public interest to do so

3.3 In the course of your professional practice you may receive requests for confidential patient information from a variety of people (for example a patient's relative, partner or carer) or organisations (for example the police or a healthcare regulator). You should make decisions about disclosing information on a case-by-case basis and fully consider all relevant factors.

3.4 If a patient with capacity refuses to give consent for information to be shared with other healthcare professionals involved in providing care, it may mean that the care they can be provided is limited. You must respect their decision, but inform the patient of the potential implications on their care or treatment.

3.5 You must respect the wishes of a patient with capacity who does not consent to information about him or her being shared with others, unless the law says you must disclose the information or it is in the public interest to make such a disclosure.

3.6 If you decide to disclose confidential patient information you should:

- code the information, or make it anonymous, if you do not need to identify the patient

- get the patient's consent to share their information. But you do not need to do this if:
  - disclosure is required by law
  - the disclosure can be justified in the public interest,
  - to do so is impracticable, would put you or others at risk of serious harm, or would prejudice the purpose of the disclosure

- disclose only the information needed for the particular purpose

- make sure that, if you disclose confidential information, the people receiving the information know that it is confidential and is to be treated as such

- make appropriate records to show:
  - who the request came from
  - whether you obtained the patient's consent, or your reasons for not doing so
  - whether consent was given or refused, and
  - what you disclosed
- be prepared to justify your decisions and any actions you take
- release the information promptly once you are satisfied what information should be disclosed and have taken all necessary steps to protect confidentiality.

3A DISCLOSING INFORMATION WITH CONSENT

3.7 You should get the patient's consent to share their information unless that would undermine the purpose of disclosure (see Section 3b).

3.8 Make sure the patient understands:
- what information will be disclosed
- why information will be disclosed
- who it will be disclosed to
- the likely consequences of disclosing and of not disclosing the information.

3.9 When the reason for sharing confidential patient information is for a purpose that the patient would not reasonably expect, you must get their explicit consent before disclosure.

3.10 If you are not sure whether you have the patient's consent to share their information, you should contact them and obtain their consent.

3B DISCLOSING INFORMATION WITHOUT CONSENT

3.11 You should make every effort to get consent to disclose confidential information. However, if that would undermine the purpose of disclosure (for example when there is risk to others) or is not practicable, you should use the guidance in this section.

3.12 Before you disclose information without the consent of the patient, you should:

- be satisfied that the law requires you to disclose the information or that disclosure can be justified as being in the public interest
- ask for clarification from the person making the request if you are unsure about the basis for the request for confidential information
- ask for the request in writing.

3.13 If necessary get advice from a relevant body, for example your indemnity insurance provider, union, professional body or other pharmacy organisation, or an independent legal advisor.

DISCLOSURES REQUIRED BY LAW

3.14 There are circumstances when the law may require you to disclose information that you hold. These circumstances include when a person or body is using their powers under the law to ask for the information, for example:
- the police or another enforcement, prosecuting or regulatory authority
- a healthcare regulator, such as ourselves or the GMC
- an NHS counter-fraud investigation officer
- a coroner or procurator fiscal, judge, or relevant court which orders that the information should be disclosed.

3.15 These individuals and organisations do not have an automatic right to access all confidential patient information. You must be satisfied they have a legitimate reason for requesting the information.

3.16 If necessary get advice from a relevant body, for example your indemnity insurance provider, union, professional body or other pharmacy organisation or an independent legal advisor.

DISCLOSURES MADE IN THE PUBLIC INTEREST

3.17 These decisions are complex and must take account of both the patient and public interest in maintaining or breaching confidentiality.

3.18 You may disclose confidential information when you consider it to be in the public interest to do so, for example if the information is required to prevent:
- a serious crime
- serious harm to a patient or third party, or
- serious risk to public health.

3.19 You must carefully balance the competing interests of maintaining the confidentiality of the information and the public interest benefit in disclosing the information.

3.20 You must consider the possible harm that may be caused by not disclosing the information against the potential consequences of disclosing the information. This includes considering how disclosing the information may affect the care of the patient and the trust that they have in pharmacy professionals.

3.21 If necessary get advice from a relevant body, for example your indemnity insurance provider, union, professional body or other pharmacy organisation, or independent legal advisor.

4 OTHER SOURCES OF INFORMATION

THE INFORMATION COMMISSIONER'S OFFICE

Phone: 0303 123 1113 or 01625 545745

HEAD OFFICE

Wycliffe House,
Water Lane,
Wilmslow,
Cheshire SK9 5AF

SCOTLAND OFFICE

45 Melville Street,
Edinburgh EH3 7HL

WALES OFFICE

2nd Floor Churchill House,
Churchill Way,
Cardiff CF10 2HH

Email: casework@ico.gsi.gov.uk

Website: www.ico.gov.uk

APPENDIX 5: GPhC GUIDANCE ON CONSENT

This guidance should be read alongside the **standards of conduct, ethics and performance** which all pharmacists and pharmacy technicians must apply to their practice. This document gives guidance on standard 3.6 of the standards of conduct, ethics and performance, which says:

You must get consent for the professional services you provide and the patient information you use.

This document gives guidance to pharmacy professionals on how to meet the standard of consent. The guidance is not intended to cover every situation and it does not give detailed legal advice. However, it reflects the current law in Great Britain.

Pharmacy professionals work in many different settings, so how relevant this guidance is to you may vary depending on your role and the type of patient contact that you have. You should use your professional judgment in applying this guidance in your own practice. You must make sure that you keep up to date and comply with the law, and with any NHS or employment policies for consent that apply to your particular area of work.

You must make sure that all staff members you are responsible for are aware of this guidance and are appropriately trained in all areas that are relevant to their duties.

If you are not sure about how the law applies in a specific situation, you should always ask for advice from appropriate professional colleagues, your employer, your professional indemnity insurance provider, your professional body or other pharmacy organisation, or get independent legal advice.

We have produced more guidance to help pharmacy professionals apply our standards of conduct, ethics and performance. You can find this on our website. In particular, when reading this guidance you should also see our 'Guidance on patient confidentiality'.

1 CONSENT

1.1 WHAT IS CONSENT?

1.1.1 The Oxford English Dictionary defines 'consent' as 'to express willingness, give permission, agree'.

1.1.2 Patients have a basic right to be involved in decisions about their healthcare. The process of obtaining consent is a fundamental part of respect for patients' rights.

1.1.3 Obtaining consent is also essential in forming and maintaining effective partnerships between you and your patients.

1.1.4 You have a professional and legal duty to get a patient's consent for the professional services, treatment or care you provide, or to use patient information.

1.1.5 You must know and comply with the law and the good practice requirements about consent which apply to you in your day-to-day practice.

1.2 TYPES OF CONSENT

1.2.1 There are two types of consent:

- explicit (or 'express') consent: when a patient gives you specific permission to do something, either spoken or written

- implied consent: when a patient indicates their consent indirectly, for example by bringing their prescription to you to be dispensed. This is not a lesser form of consent but it is only valid if the patient knows and understands what they are consenting to. If you are not sure whether you have implied consent, you should get explicit consent.

1.2.2 You must use your professional judgment to decide what type of consent to get. You should take into account legal requirements, NHS service requirements, and policies where you work that may set this out.

1.2.3 When appropriate, you should record the fact that the patient has given explicit consent and what they have consented to.

1.3 OBTAINING CONSENT

1.3.1 For consent to be valid the patient must:
- have the capacity to give consent
- be acting voluntarily – they must not be under any undue pressure from you or anyone else to make a decision
- have sufficient, balanced information to allow them to make an informed decision
- be capable of using and weighing up the information provided.

1.3.2 The information you provide to the patient must be clear, accurate and presented in a way that the patient can understand. For example, you must consider any disabilities, or literacy or language barriers.

1.3.3 You should not make assumptions about the patient's level of knowledge and you should give them the opportunity to ask questions.

1.3.4 You are responsible for making sure that a patient has given valid consent. You must use your professional judgment to decide whether you should get consent from the patient yourself, or whether this task can be properly delegated. If you do delegate the task you must make sure that you delegate it to a competent and appropriately trained member of staff.

1.3.5 Getting consent is an ongoing process between you and the patient. Consent cannot be presumed just because it was given on a previous occasion. You must get a patient's consent on each occasion that it is needed, for example when there is a change in treatment or service options.

1.3.6 Patients with capacity are entitled to withdraw their consent at any time.

2 CAPACITY

2.1 WHAT IS CAPACITY?

2.1.1 In England and Wales, under the Mental Capacity Act (2005), a person lacks capacity if at the time the decision needs to be made, they are unable to make or communicate the decision, because of an 'impairment or disturbance' that affects the way their mind or brain works.

2.1.2 In Scotland, under the Adults with Incapacity (Scotland) Act (2000), a person lacks capacity if they cannot make decisions or communicate them, or understand or remember their decisions, because of a mental disorder or physical inability to communicate in any form.

2.2 ASSESSING CAPACITY

2.2.1 You must base an assessment of capacity on the patient's ability to make a specific decision at the time it needs to be made. A patient may be capable of making some decisions but not others.

2.2.2 In general, to make an informed decision the patient should be able to:
- understand the information provided
- remember the information provided
- use and weigh up the information provided, and
- communicate their decision to you (by any means).

2.2.3 You must not assume that because a patient lacks capacity on one occasion, or in relation to one type of service, that they lack capacity to make all decisions.

2.2.4 A patient's capacity to consent may be temporarily affected by other factors, for example fatigue, panic, or the effects of drugs or alcohol. The existence of these factors should not lead to an automatic assumption that the patient does not have the capacity to consent. Instead you should use your professional judgment to make a decision based on the individual circumstances.

2.2.5 You must not assume that a patient lacks capacity based just upon their age, disability, beliefs, condition, or behaviour, or because they make a decision you disagree with.

2.2.6 You must take all reasonable steps to help and support patients to make their own decisions or to be as involved as they can be in a decision. For example:
- time the discussion for when the patient's understanding may be better
- use appropriate types of communication, simple language or visual aids
- get someone else to help with communication such as a family member, support worker or interpreter.

2.2.7 If you are unsure about a patient's capacity you must get advice from other healthcare professionals or people involved in their care.

2.2.8 If you are still unsure you must get legal advice.

2.2.9 Any advice you get or assessments carried out should be properly recorded, along with the outcome.

2.2.10 You can find more guidance on how people should be helped to make their own decisions, and how to assess capacity, in the Codes of Practice that accompany the Mental Capacity Act (2005) and Adults with Incapacity (Scotland) Act (2000).

2.3 ADULTS WITH CAPACITY

2.3.1 Every adult is presumed to have the capacity to make their own decisions (that is, they are competent) and to give consent for a service or treatment unless there is enough evidence to suggest otherwise.

2.4 WHEN A COMPETENT ADULT REFUSES TO GIVE CONSENT

2.4.1 If an adult with capacity makes a voluntary, informed decision to refuse a service or treatment you must respect their decision, even when you think that their decision is wrong or may cause them harm. This does not apply when the law says otherwise, such as when compulsory treatment is authorised by mental health legislation[1].

2.4.2 You should clearly explain the consequences of their decision but you must make sure that you do not pressure the patient to accept your advice.

2.4.3 You should make a detailed record if a patient refuses to give consent. This should include the discussions that have taken place and the advice you gave.

2.4.4 If you believe that the patient is at risk of serious harm due to their decision to refuse a service or treatment, you must raise this issue with appropriate healthcare or pharmacy colleagues or people involved in their care, and your employer (if applicable). Consider getting legal advice if necessary.

1 Mental Health Act 2003 (as amended by the Mental Health Act 2006), and the Mental Health (Care and Treatment) (Scotland) Act 2003.

2.5 ADULTS WITHOUT CAPACITY

2.5.1 If the patient is not able to make decisions for themselves, you must work with people close to them and with other members of the healthcare team.

2.5.2 The Mental Capacity Act (2005) and Adults with Incapacity (Scotland) Act (2000) set out the criteria and the processes to be followed in making decisions and providing care services when a patient lacks the capacity to make some or all decisions for themselves. They also grant legal authority to certain people to make decisions on behalf of patients who lack capacity.

2.5.3 If you believe that a patient lacks capacity to make decisions for themselves, consult the Codes of Practice that accompany the Mental Capacity Act (2005) or Adults with Incapacity (Scotland) Act (2000). These set out who can make decisions on the patient's behalf, in which situations, and how they should go about this.

2.6 YOUNG PEOPLE AND CHILDREN

2.6.1 The capacity to consent depends more on the patient's ability to understand and consider their decision than on their age.

2.6.2 In this guidance a young person means anyone aged 16 or 17 and a child means anyone aged under 16. However, people gain full legal capacity in relation to medical treatment at a different age in Scotland than in England and Wales.

2.6.3 As with any patient, a young person or child may have the capacity to consent to some services or treatments but not to others. Therefore it is important that you assess maturity and understanding individually, and bearing in mind the complexity and importance of the decision to be made.

2.6.4 If a person with parental responsibility is required to provide consent, you may need to get legal advice if:

- you are in any doubt about who has parental responsibility for the individual, or
- the views of those that have parental responsibility differ.

2.6.5 Young people and children should be involved as much as possible in decisions about their care, even when they are not able to make decisions on their own.

2.7 YOUNG PEOPLE WITH CAPACITY

2.7.1 Young people are presumed to have the capacity to make their own decisions and give consent for a service or treatment, unless there is enough evidence to suggest otherwise.

2.7.2 To decide whether a young person has the capacity to consent to a service or treatment, use the same criteria as for adults (see section 2.2 'Assessing capacity').

2.7.3 You should encourage young people to involve their parents in making important decisions. However, you should respect a competent young person's request for confidentiality.

2.8 CHILDREN WITH CAPACITY

2.8.1 Children are not presumed to have the capacity to consent. They must demonstrate their competence.

2.8.2 A child can give consent if you are satisfied that the treatment is in their best interests, and that they have the maturity and ability to fully understand the information given and what they are consenting to. In this case you do not also need consent from a person with parental responsibility.

2.9 WHEN COMPETENT YOUNG PEOPLE AND CHILDREN REFUSE TO GIVE CONSENT

England and Wales

2.9.1 In some circumstances, the courts can override the refusal of consent of a young person or child. You should get legal advice if needed on this issue.

2.9.2 The law is complex when a competent young person or child refuses to give consent for a treatment or service and someone with parental responsibility wants to override their decision. You should get legal advice if you are faced with this situation.

Scotland

2.9.3 When a young person or child has capacity to make a decision, then the law[2] says that their decision should be respected. This applies even if the decision differs from your view, or from the views of those with parental responsibility.

2.9.4 However, this position has not yet been fully tested in the Scottish courts, and nor has the issue of whether a court can override a young person's or child's decision. You should therefore get legal advice if you are faced with this situation.

2 The Age of Legal Capacity (Scotland) Act 1991.

2.10 YOUNG PEOPLE WITHOUT CAPACITY

England and Wales

2.10.1 A person with parental responsibility for a young person can give consent on behalf of that young person to investigations and treatment that are in the young person's best interests.

Scotland

2.10.2 The rights of a person with parental responsibility to make decisions on behalf of a child ends when the child reaches the age of 16.

2.10.3 Young people who do not have the capacity to consent should be treated as though they are adults and in line with the Adults with Incapacity (Scotland) Act (2000).

2.11 CHILDREN WITHOUT CAPACITY

2.11.1 When a child lacks capacity to give consent, any person with parental responsibility for that child, or the court, can give consent on their behalf.

3 ADVANCE DECISIONS

3.1 People who understand the implications of their choices can say in advance how they want to be treated if they later suffer loss of mental capacity.

3.2 An unambiguous advance refusal for a treatment, procedure or intervention which is voluntarily made by a competent, informed adult is likely to have legal force.

3.3 An advance refusal of treatment cannot override the legal authority to give compulsory treatment under the mental health laws.

3.4 Any advance decision is superseded by a competent decision by the person concerned, given at the time consent is sought.

England and Wales

3.5 Advance decisions are covered by the Mental Capacity Act (2005). For an advance refusal of treatment to be legally valid, it must meet certain criteria set out in the Mental Capacity Act (2005).

3.6   If an advance decision does not meet these criteria, it is not legally binding but can still be used in deciding the patient's best interests.

3.7   You must follow an advance decision if it is valid and applicable to current circumstances.

Scotland

3.8   The Adults with Incapacity (Scotland) Act (2000) does not specifically cover advance decisions. However, it says that health professionals must take account of the patient's past and present wishes, however they were communicated.

3.9   It is likely that you would be bound by a valid and applicable advance decision. However, there have been no specific cases yet considered by the Scottish courts. If in any doubt, get legal advice.

4 EMERGENCIES

4.1   In an emergency, if you cannot get consent, you can provide treatment that is in the patient's best interests and is needed to save their life or prevent deterioration in the patient's condition (this applies to children, young people and adults).

4.2   There is an exception to 4.1 above if you know there is a valid and applicable advance decision to refuse a particular treatment. For more information see the relevant incapacity legislation and its Code of Practice, or ask your professional indemnity insurance provider or a legal advisor.

5 OTHER SOURCES OF INFORMATION

ENGLAND AND WALES

Mental Capacity Act 2005

www.legislation.gov.uk/ukpga/2005/9/contents

Mental Capacity Act Code of Practice

www.publicguardian.gov.uk/mca/code-of-practice.htm

SCOTLAND

Adults with Incapacity (Scotland) Act 2000

www.legislation.gov.uk/asp/2000/4/contents

Scottish Government site for the Act

www.scotland.gov.uk/Topics/Justice/Civil/awi

APPENDICES

APPENDIX 6: GPhC GUIDANCE ON RAISING CONCERNS

The issue of raising concerns has been the subject of several high-profile cases in the past twenty years, including the inquiry into Bristol Royal Infirmary and the Shipman Inquiry. The Health Select Committee highlighted in two public reports[1] the importance of healthcare professionals raising concerns. It is therefore important to give pharmacists and pharmacy technicians guidance on this subject. We must make sure that we all learn from past incidents and the experiences of other regulators.

This guidance should be read alongside the **standards of conduct, ethics and performance** which all pharmacists and pharmacy technicians must apply to their practice.

This document gives guidance on standards 1.2, 2.4 and 7.11 of the standards of conduct, ethics and performance, which say:

- You must take action to protect the well-being of patients and the public.

- You must be prepared to challenge the judgment of your colleagues and other professionals if you have reason to believe that their decisions could affect the safety or care of others.

- You must make the relevant authority aware of any policies, systems, working conditions, or the actions, professional performance, or health of others if they may affect patient care or public safety. If something goes wrong or if someone reports a concern to you, make sure that you deal with it appropriately.

This document gives guidance to pharmacy professionals on how to raise concerns. The guidance explains the importance of raising concerns and the steps that a pharmacy professional will need to consider taking.

It also contains extra guidance specifically for employers. You can find the contact details of organisations that may be able to give further support and guidance in section 6 of this document.

You must make sure that you keep up to date with and follow any NHS or employment policies for raising concerns where you practise. You must also make sure that all staff members you are responsible for are aware of this guidance and appropriately trained.

1 THE IMPORTANCE OF RAISING CONCERNS

Every pharmacy professional has a duty to raise any concerns about individuals, actions or circumstances that may be unacceptable and that could result in risks to patient and public safety.

1.1 You have a professional responsibility to take action to protect the wellbeing of patients and the public. Raising concerns about individual pharmacy professionals, the staff you work with (including trainees), employers and the environment you work in is a key part of this.

1.2 This includes raising and reporting any concerns you have about the people you come into contact with during the course of your work, including pharmacists, pharmacy technicians, pharmacy owners, managers and employers, other healthcare professionals or people responsible for the care of a patient, such as carers, care home staff or key workers. It includes concerns about behaviours, competency, the working environment and any actions that may compromise patient safety.

1.3 We recognise that you may be reluctant to raise a concern for a variety of reasons. For example, you may be worried that:

- you will cause trouble for your colleagues
- there may be a negative impact on your career
- it may lead to difficult working relationships with your colleagues
- you could face reprisals
- nothing will be done as a result of the concern being raised.

Raising concerns at an early stage can help to identify areas of practice that can be improved. It allows employers, regulators and other authorities to take corrective action as quickly as possible and before any direct harm comes to patients and the public.

1.4 You must remember that:

- your professional duties to safeguard patient and public safety must come before any other loyalties or considerations

- failing to raise concerns about poor practice could result in harm to patients

- the Public Interest Disclosure Act 1998 (PIDA) protects employees who raise genuine concerns and expose 'malpractice' in the workplace

- if you do not report any concerns you may have about a colleague or others it would be a breach of our standards of conduct, ethics and performance, and this may call into question your own fitness to practise.

2 HOW TO RAISE A CONCERN

How you raise a concern will vary, depending on:

- The nature of your concern
- Who or what you are concerned about, and
- Whether you consider there is a direct or immediate risk of harm to patients or the public.

If you are not sure whether or how to raise your concern you should get advice from one of the organisations listed in section 6.

You have a professional responsibility to raise genuine concerns. You have this responsibility whether you are an employer, employee, a locum or temporary staff.

You should normally raise your concern with your employer first, before taking it to a regulator or other organisation.

2.1 FIND OUT YOUR ORGANISATION'S POLICY
You should find out your employer's policy on raising concerns or 'whistle blowing' and follow this whenever possible.

2.2 REPORT WITHOUT DELAY
If you believe that patients are or may be at risk of death or serious harm you must report your concern without delay.

2.3 REPORT TO YOUR IMMEDIATE SUPERVISOR
The person you report your concerns to will vary depending on the nature of your concern. In most situations, you will be able to raise your concerns with your line manager.

2.4 REPORT TO ANOTHER SUITABLE PERSON IN AUTHORITY OR AN OUTSIDE BODY
There may be some situations when it isn't possible to raise your concerns with your line manager. For example, they may be the cause of your concern or may have strong loyalties to those who are the cause of your concern. In these situations, you may need to speak to:

- a person who has been named as responsible for handling concerns

- a senior manager in the organisation, for example a chief pharmacist, pharmacy owner or superintendent pharmacist or non-pharmacist manager

- the primary care organisation (including the accountable officer if the concern is about controlled drugs)

- the health or social care profession regulator[2]

- the relevant systems regulator for the organisation[3].

2.5 KEEP A RECORD
You should keep a record of the concerns you have, who you have raised them with and the response or action that has been taken as a result of your actions.

2.6 MAINTAIN CONFIDENTIALITY
If your concern is about a specific person, for example a patient or colleague, you should, where possible, maintain confidentiality and not disclose information without consent.

3 THE LAW

The PIDA sets out a step-by-step approach to raising and escalating your concern. It aims to protect you from unfair treatment or victimization from your employer if you have made certain disclosures of information in the public interest.

Under the PIDA you should raise a concern about issues which have happened, or which you reasonably believe are likely to happen, and involve:

- A danger to the health or safety of an individual (for example, irresponsible or illegal prescribing, patient abuse, or a professional whose health or fitness to practise may be impaired)

- A crime, or a civil offence (for example, fraud, theft, or the illegal diversion of drugs)
- A miscarriage of justice
- Damage to the environment
- A cover-up of information about any of the above.

This is not a full list. Section 6 gives contact details for other sources of information if you have a concern and you are unsure about whether or how you should raise it.

4 EXTRA GUIDANCE FOR EMPLOYERS

It is important that employees know about the procedures to follow if they have a concern about a colleague or the organisation they work in.

There should also be procedures to identify concerns that should be referred to a regulatory body such as ourselves. Creating an open working environment where your employees feel comfortable raising concerns will safeguard patient safety by helping to identify and therefore improve poor practice.

4.1 Make sure you have fair and robust policies and procedures to manage concerns that are raised with you. These policies and procedures need to be accessible to all staff.

4.2 Encourage all staff, including temporary staff and locums, to raise concerns about the safety of patients, including risks posed by colleagues.

4.3 Make sure that all concerns raised with you are taken seriously and the person who has raised them is not victimised.

4.4 Make sure that all concerns are properly investigated and that all staff, including temporary staff and locums, are kept informed of the progress.

4.5 Have systems in place to give adequate support to pharmacy professionals who have raised concerns, and treat any information you are given in confidence.

4.6 Take appropriate steps to deal with concerns that have been raised because of a failure to maintain standards.

4.7 Have systems in place to support pharmacy professionals who are the subject of the concern, whether it is due to their poor performance, health or behaviour.

4.8 Keep appropriate records of any concerns raised and the actions taken to deal with them.

4.9 Pass records of concerns raised to the manager or superintendent pharmacist so that they can consider an overall assessment of the concerns.

4.10 Do not stop anyone from raising a concern.

5 WHERE TO GO FOR MORE ADVICE

For more information on the PIDA and how to raise your concern under this employment legislation you may want to contact the charity Public Concern at Work (PCaW). This is an independent charity that gives free, confidential legal advice to people who are not sure whether or how to raise concerns about 'malpractice' at work.

If you are not sure whether or how to raise your concern you should get advice from:

- Senior members of staff in your organisation
- The accountable officer, if the concern is about controlled drugs
- Your professional indemnity insurance provider, professional body or other pharmacy organisation
- The General Pharmaceutical Council or, if your concern is about a colleague in another healthcare profession, the appropriate regulatory body
- The charity Pharmacist Support
- Your union
- An independent legal advisor.

6 OTHER SOURCES OF INFORMATION

ASSOCIATION OF PHARMACY TECHNICIANS UK

One Victoria Square,
Birmingham, B1 1BD
Phone: 020 7121 5551

www.aptuk.org

GUILD OF HEALTHCARE PHARMACISTS

Health Sector, Unite the Union,
Unite House, 126 Theobald's Road,
London, WC1X 8TN
Phone: 0203 371 2009

www.ghp.org.uk
www.ghpscot.org.uk

NATIONAL PHARMACY ASSOCIATION

Mallinson House, 38-42 St Peter's Street,
St Albans AL1 3NP

Phone: 01727 858687

www.npa.co.uk

NATIONAL WHISTLEBLOWING HELPLINE

Phone: 08000 724 725

PHARMACISTS' DEFENCE ASSOCIATION

The Old Fire Station, 69 Albion Street,
Birmingham B1 3EA

Phone: 0121 694 7000

www.the-pda.org

PHARMACIST SUPPORT

Phone: 0808 168 2233 (freephone)

www.pharmacistsupport.org

PUBLIC CONCERN AT WORK

Suite 301, 16 Baldwins Gardens,
London EC1N 7RJ

Phone: 020 7404 6609

www.pcaw.co.uk

ROYAL PHARMACEUTICAL SOCIETY

1 Lambeth High Street, London SE1 7JN

Phone: 0845 257 2570

www.rpharms.com

UNISON

UNISON Centre, 130 Euston Road,
London NW1 2AY

Phone: 0845 355 0845

www.unison.org.uk

1 http://www.parliament.uk/business/committees/committees-a-z/commons-select/healthcommittee/news/11-07-26-nmcreportpublished/

2 The healthcare regulators are: General Chiropractic Council; General Dental Council; General Medical Council; General Optical Council; General Osteopathic Council; Health Professions Council; Nursing and Midwifery Council; General Pharmaceutical Council and Pharmaceutical Society of Northern Ireland. The social care regulators are the Care Council in Wales; General Social Care Council in England; Northern Ireland Social Care Council and the Scottish Social Services Council.

3 These include, within the hospital setting, the Care Quality Commission in England, the Health Inspectorate Wales, Healthcare Improvement Scotland and the General Pharmaceutical Council if the concern is about registered pharmacy premises.

APPENDIX 7: GPhC GUIDANCE ON MAINTAINING CLEAR SEXUAL BOUNDARIES

This guidance should be read alongside the standards of conduct, ethics and performance which all pharmacists and pharmacy technicians must apply to their practice. This document gives guidance on standard 3.9 of the standards of conduct, ethics and performance, which says:

You must maintain proper professional boundaries in your relationships with patients and others you come into contact with during the course of your professional practice and take special care when dealing with vulnerable people.

This document gives guidance to pharmacy professionals on the importance of maintaining clear sexual boundaries, and explains the responsibilities pharmacy professionals have. We have based this guidance on the Council for Healthcare Regulatory Excellence (CHRE) document **'Clear sexual boundaries between healthcare professionals and patients: responsibilities of healthcare professionals'**[1].

You must make sure that all staff members you are responsible for are aware of this guidance and appropriately trained in all areas that are relevant to their duties.

If you are not sure about what you should do in a specific situation, you should always ask for advice from your employer, professional indemnity insurance provider, professional body or other pharmacy organisation, or get independent legal advice.

*1 CHRE: Clear sexual boundaries between healthcare professionals and patients: responsibilities of healthcare professionals: **www.chre.org.uk***

1 WHY IT'S IMPORTANT TO MAINTAIN CLEAR SEXUAL BOUNDARIES

1.1 When healthcare professionals cross professional boundaries the result for patients can be serious and can cause lasting harm. If you cross these boundaries it can damage public trust and confidence in the pharmacy profession and other healthcare professions.

1.2 Patients must be able to trust that you will act in their best interests. If you are sexually, or inappropriately, involved with a patient, your professional judgment can be affected. This involvement may affect the decisions that you make about their healthcare.

2 POWER IMBALANCE

2.1 The CHRE document explains that 'an imbalance of power is often a feature in the healthcare professional/patient relationship, although this may not be explicit'.

2.2 Patients are often vulnerable when they need healthcare. In the relationship between a patient and a healthcare professional, there is often a power imbalance. This may be because the patient shares personal information with you or because you have information and resources (such as medicines) that the patient needs. The patient may not be familiar with the situation they are in, or know what is appropriate professional behaviour. Therefore they may not be able to properly judge that the patient/professional relationship, or what happens to them, is appropriate. It is your responsibility to be aware of the imbalance of power and to maintain clear boundaries at all times.

2.3　You should always be clear with the patient about the reason for an examination or why you want them to come into the consultation room. Give them all the information they need and the opportunity to ask questions, and get their consent before going ahead.

3 SEXUALISED BEHAVIOUR AND BREACHES OF SEXUAL BOUNDARIES

3.1　The CHRE document defines sexualised behaviour as 'acts, words or behaviour designed to arouse or gratify sexual impulses or desires'.

3.2　A breach of sexual boundaries is not limited to criminal acts, such as rape or sexual assault. For example, carrying out an unnecessary physical examination or asking for details of sexual orientation when it is not necessary or relevant, would both be a breach.

4 AVOIDING BREACHES OF SEXUAL BOUNDARIES

4.1　There are a number of behaviours that may be signs of showing sexualised behaviour towards patients or carers. These include:

- when the healthcare professional reveals intimate personal details about themselves to a patient during a consultation
- when the reason behind the following actions is sexual:
  - giving or accepting social invitations (dates and meetings)
  - visiting a patient's home without an appointment
  - meeting patients outside of normal practice, for example arranging appointments for a time when no other staff are in the pharmacy
  - asking questions unrelated to the patient's health.

4.2　If you find yourself in a situation where you are attracted to a patient, you must not act on these feelings. If you have concerns that this may affect your professional judgment, or if you are not sure whether you are abusing your professional position, you may find it helpful to discuss this with someone else.
You might discuss this with an impartial colleague, a pharmacy organisation that represents you, a professional leadership body or your professional indemnity insurance provider.

4.3　If you cannot continue to care for the patient and be objective, you should find other care for the patient. You must make sure there is a proper handover to another pharmacy professional and that the patient does not feel that they are in the wrong as a result of your actions.

4.4　There may be situations when patients or their carers are attracted to you. If a patient shows sexualised behaviour towards you, you should think about whether you should discuss their feelings in a constructive way and try to re-establish a professional relationship. If this is not possible, you should transfer the patient's care to another pharmacy professional. You may find it helpful to discuss the matter with a colleague, a pharmacy organisation that represents you, a professional leadership body or your professional indemnity insurance provider.

5 CHAPERONES

5.1　A chaperone is a person (usually the same sex as the patient) who is present as a safeguard for the patient and the healthcare professional. They are also a witness to the patient's continuing consent for the procedure. Their role may vary depending on the needs of the patient, the pharmacy professional and the examination or procedure being carried out.

5.2　You should ask the patient whether they would like a chaperone to be with them in the consultation room, and for any examination that they might consider to be intimate. You should discuss the need for a chaperone with the patient and should not guess what their wishes are.

5.3 You should record any discussion that you have with patients about chaperones, including when the patient says that they do not want to have a chaperone present.

5.4 If no chaperone is available you should offer to delay and re-arrange the consultation or examination until one is available (unless a delay is not in the patient's best interests).

6 CULTURAL AND OTHER DIFFERENCES

6.1 Cultural differences can affect a patient's view of their personal boundaries and what is appropriate. You need to be sensitive to this, and always treat patients as individuals in a way that respects their views and maintains their dignity. For example, an individual may prefer to talk to or be examined by a pharmacy professional of the same gender, or have another person present.

7 PREVIOUS PATIENTS OR CARERS

7.1 The same principles apply to patients or carers that you have dealt with in the past and are not your patients any more. The previous professional relationship may also have involved an imbalance of power, and so would affect any personal relationship. If you think that this type of relationship may develop, you should consider the consequences or any harm this may cause to the patient and the impact on your professional standing. We advise you to consider the following:

- how long the professional relationship lasted and when it ended

- the nature of the previous professional relationship and whether it involved a significant imbalance of power

- whether the former patient or carer was, or is, vulnerable

- whether you are using the knowledge or influence that you gained through the professional relationship to develop or continue the personal relationship

- whether you are already treating, or are likely to treat, any other members of the former patient's or carer's family.

7.2 It is your responsibility as a pharmacy professional to act appropriately and professionally, even if the relationship is agreed by everyone involved. You must consider all the issues above and, if necessary, get appropriate advice.

8 RAISING CONCERNS

8.1 You have a professional duty to raise concerns if you believe the actions of other individuals are putting patients at risk. This would include when you are concerned that clear sexual boundaries have not been maintained by other healthcare professionals. You must also take appropriate action if others report concerns to you.

8.2 See our document 'Guidance on raising concerns' for more information.

9 OTHER USEFUL SOURCES OF INFORMATION

- Clear sexual boundaries between healthcare professionals and patients: responsibilities of healthcare professionals, CHRE: **www.chre.org.uk**

- Chaperone Framework, PSNC: **www.psnc.org.uk**

APPENDIX 8: GPhC GUIDANCE ON THE PROVISION OF PHARMACY SERVICES AFFECTED BY RELIGIOUS AND MORAL BELIEFS

The General Pharmaceutical Council is the regulator for pharmacists, pharmacy technicians and registered pharmacy premises in England, Scotland and Wales. As part of our role, we set the standards which govern the practice of pharmacists and pharmacy technicians.

This document provides guidance on standard 3.4 of the standards of conduct, ethics and performance which states:

You must make sure that if your religious or moral beliefs prevent you from providing a service, you tell the relevant people or authorities and refer patients and the public to other providers.

This document gives guidance to pharmacy professionals on what they need to do if their religious or moral beliefs affect the provision of pharmacy services to patients and the public. Pharmacy professionals may also need to consider their contractual obligations, such as the NHS Terms of Service, if they are unable to provide a service.

This document also provides guidance to employers on what they need to do if they employ a pharmacy professional whose religious or moral beliefs may affect a service they provide.

NB: The GPhC has agreed that this provision will be reviewed during the first 12 months of operation.

GUIDANCE FOR PHARMACY PROFESSIONALS

Failure to provide specific pharmacy services will affect patients and the public, colleagues, employers and service commissioners. It is essential that relevant persons are informed and that patients and the public are directed to other service providers.

If your beliefs prevent you from providing a pharmacy service you should:

BEFORE ACCEPTING EMPLOYMENT

1.1 Think about where you are going to work and if the services you object to providing will be available and accessible in that vicinity. You need to remember that you must make patients your first concern

1.2 Find out:
- if you will be working on your own or with other pharmacy professionals who will be able to provide the service
- where you would direct patients requesting the service
- whether the service you intend to direct patients to will be accessible and readily available to them at the time you will be on duty

1.3 Tell employers, relevant authorities and the colleagues you will be working with about your beliefs. The persons or authorities who need to be informed may include:
- the superintendent pharmacist, pharmacy owner, pharmacist manager or other person responsible for employing pharmacists
- locum agencies from whom you are seeking employment
- the primary care organisation or other body with whom you or the owner has a contract for services

RESPONDING TO REQUESTS FOR A SERVICE

1.4 You are responsible for ensuring that the patient is properly informed about why the service they are requesting is not available. Be open and honest about your reasons for not providing a service as this will help patients understand and maintain trust and confidence in the profession

1.5 Handle the situation sensitively. In some cases the initial request for a service will be made to another member of the pharmacy team so make sure that all staff are aware of your views and are trained to deal with the initial requests for services affected by your beliefs

1.6 Respect the patient's right to confidentiality and take all reasonable steps to ensure appropriate levels of privacy for patient consultations even when you are unable to provide a service

1.7 Patients should not be discouraged from seeking further information or advice. Remember:

- if you do not supply emergency hormonal contraception (EHC) (either over the counter or against a prescription), women should be referred to an alternative appropriate source of supply available within the time limits for EHC to be effective

- if you do not supply routine hormonal contraception, women should be referred to an alternative appropriate source of supply available within the time period which will not compromise the woman's contraceptive cover

- if you refer a patient to a doctor's surgery or hospital you should think about whether the patient will be seen by a doctor or other appropriate practitioner within the timeframe required for treatment to be effective (i.e. consider factors such as the practice's opening hours and whether the patient will be able to get there)

- if you refer a patient to another pharmacy, check that there will be a pharmacist available there who can provide the service and that they have the relevant stock

GUIDANCE FOR EMPLOYERS

Before you employ a pharmacy professional check whether they have any beliefs that prevent them from providing a particular pharmacy service. You must consider whether patients could be directed to alternative providers of the affected service in the vicinity. When you employ pharmacy professionals whose beliefs prevent them from providing a pharmacy service, you should:

2.1 Be satisfied that enough information has been given to the pharmacy professional about the services provided in the pharmacy they are going to work in

2.2 Have policies and procedures to guide staff in managing requests for services affected by moral and religious beliefs so that requests are handled appropriately and patients are able to access the services they require. Clear information on alternative services must be provided

2.3 Ensure staff members are appropriately trained and provide them with the contact details and availability of local providers of the affected services

APPENDIX 9: GPhC GUIDANCE FOR OWNERS AND SUPERINTENDENT PHARMACISTS WHO EMPLOY RESPONSIBLE PHARMACISTS

The General Pharmaceutical Council is the regulator for pharmacists, pharmacy technicians and registered pharmacy premises in England, Scotland and Wales. As part of our role, we set the standards which govern the practice of pharmacists and pharmacy technicians.

This document provides guidance on the standards for pharmacy owners and superintendent pharmacists of retail pharmacy businesses in relation to the responsible pharmacist regulations.

This document gives guidance to owners and superintendent pharmacists on what they need to do when they employ a responsible pharmacist.

This guidance only relates to your responsibilities as a pharmacy owner or superintendent pharmacist in relation to the responsible pharmacist regulations and does not cover your other duties and obligations.

This document does not give legal advice and you must ensure that you comply with the relevant legislative requirements set out in:

- The Medicines Act 1968

- The Medicines (Pharmacies) (Responsible Pharmacist) Regulations 2008

- Any contractual obligations, such as the NHS Terms of Service

APPOINTING AND SUPPORTING THE RESPONSIBLE PHARMACIST

In order to lawfully conduct a retail pharmacy business, a registered pharmacist must be in charge of the registered pharmacy as the responsible pharmacist.

YOU MUST:

1.1 Ensure that arrangements are in place to appoint a responsible pharmacist to be in charge of each registered pharmacy for which you are the owner or superintendent pharmacist. A pharmacist can only be the responsible pharmacist in charge of one registered pharmacy at any one time

1.2 Ensure that arrangements are in place so that only a registered pharmacist who is competent and able to secure the safe and effective running of the registered pharmacy is appointed as the responsible pharmacist

1.3 Ensure that the overarching operational framework for the registered pharmacy is established

1.4 Support the responsible pharmacist in complying with their legal and professional duty to secure the safe and effective running of the registered pharmacy

1.5 Enable the responsible pharmacist to comply with their legal and professional duty to secure the safe and effective running of the registered pharmacy. This includes allowing the responsible pharmacist to exercise their professional judgment

THE PHARMACY RECORD

The pharmacy record is an important legal document. It shows who the responsible pharmacist is on any given date and at any time. This audit trail is particularly important in the event of any incident or error as it shows who was accountable. The pharmacy record may be kept in writing, electronically or in both forms. An entry in the pharmacy record may be made remotely as long as the record complies with all the relevant professional and legal requirements.

YOU MUST:

2.1   Ensure that the responsible pharmacist maintains the pharmacy record

2.2   Ensure that the pharmacy record is kept for at least five years. For electronic records this is five years from the day the record was created. For written records this is five years from the last day to which the record relates

2.3   Ensure that appropriate measures are in place to ensure that:

- the record is backed-up

- the record is available at the premises for inspection

- any alterations to the record identify when, and by whom, the alteration was made,

if the pharmacy record is maintained electronically

2.4   Ensure that the pharmacy record is available at the registered pharmacy for inspection by the responsible pharmacist, the pharmacy staff and our Inspectorate

APPENDIX 10: GPhC GUIDANCE FOR RESPONSIBLE PHARMACISTS

The General Pharmaceutical Council is the regulator for pharmacists, pharmacy technicians and registered pharmacy premises in England, Scotland and Wales. As part of our role, we set the standards which govern the practice of pharmacists and pharmacy technicians.

This document provides guidance on standard 7.7 of the standards of conduct, ethics and performance which states:

You must make sure that you keep to your legal and professional responsibilities and that your workload or working conditions do not present a risk to patient care or public safety.

This document gives guidance to pharmacists on what they need to do if they are going to take on the role as the responsible pharmacist in charge of a registered pharmacy.

This document does not give legal advice and you must ensure that you comply with the relevant legislative requirements set out in:

- The Medicines Act 1968
- The Medicines (Pharmacies) (Responsible Pharmacist) Regulations 2008
- Any contractual obligations, such as the NHS Terms of Service

SECURING THE SAFE AND EFFECTIVE RUNNING OF THE REGISTERED PHARMACY

In order to lawfully conduct a retail pharmacy business, a registered pharmacist must be in charge of the registered pharmacy as the responsible pharmacist.

The operational activities that may take place in the registered pharmacy when you are in charge of the pharmacy depend on the level of supervision provided and whether or not you are absent from the registered pharmacy. Examples of operational activities and the level of supervision required can be found in Appendix A.

YOU MUST:

1.1   Establish the scope of the role and responsibilities you will have as the responsible pharmacist and

take all reasonable steps to clarify any ambiguities or uncertainties with the pharmacy owner, superintendent pharmacist or other delegated person

1.2   Only take on the role of the responsible pharmacist if this is within your professional competence

1.3   Only be the responsible pharmacist in charge of one registered pharmacy at any given time

1.4   Secure the safe and effective running of the pharmacy business at the registered pharmacy in question before the pharmacy can undertake operational activities. Only after you are personally satisfied that you have secured the safe and effective running of the pharmacy can any operational activities begin to take place (see Appendix A).

DISPLAYING THE NOTICE

The notice is important as it allows patients and the public to identify the pharmacist who is responsible for the safe and effective running of the registered pharmacy. The details of the information that must be included on the notice can be found in Appendix B.

YOU MUST:

2.1   Conspicuously display a notice in the registered pharmacy

THE PHARMACY RECORD

The pharmacy record is an important legal document. It shows who the responsible pharmacist is on any given date and at any time. This audit trail is particularly important in the event of any incident or error as it shows who was accountable.

The pharmacy record may be kept in writing, electronically or in both forms. An entry in the pharmacy record may be made remotely as long as the record complies with all the relevant professional and legal requirements.

The details that must be recorded in the pharmacy record are provided in Appendix C.

YOU MUST:

3.1 Ensure the pharmacy record is accurate and reflects who the responsible pharmacist is, and was, at any given date and time (including whether or not the responsible pharmacist is, or was, absent from the registered pharmacy)

3.2 Personally make the entries in the pharmacy record

3.3 Ensure any amendments or alterations identify when, and by whom, the alteration was made, if the pharmacy record is maintained as a paper-based record

3.4 Be satisfied that appropriate measures are in place to ensure that:

- the record is backed-up
- the record is available at the registered pharmacy for inspection
- any alterations to the record identify when, and by whom, the alteration was made,

if the pharmacy record is maintained electronically

3.5 Not become the responsible pharmacist or make an entry in the pharmacy record until you have secured the safe and effective running of the pharmacy business at the registered pharmacy in question

3.6 Ensure that the pharmacy record is available at the registered pharmacy

3.7 Ensure that the pharmacy record is available for inspection by the person who owns the pharmacy business, the superintendent pharmacist (in the case of a body corporate), the responsible pharmacist, the pharmacy staff and our Inspectorate.

PHARMACY PROCEDURES

The pharmacy procedures form part of the quality framework for the safe and effective running of the registered pharmacy. The pharmacy procedures may be maintained in writing, electronically or in both forms.

The matters that must be covered by the pharmacy procedures are provided in Appendix D.

YOU MUST:

4.1 Establish, if not already established, maintain and review pharmacy procedures

4.2 Maintain adequate back-ups of the content of pharmacy procedures

4.3 Ensure that the pharmacy procedures are available for inspection by the person who owns the pharmacy business, the superintendent pharmacist (in the case of a body corporate), the responsible pharmacist, the pharmacy staff and our Inspectorate

4.4 Ensure that the pharmacy staff understand the pharmacy procedures that are in use

4.5 Ensure that the pharmacy procedures:

- are reviewed at least once every two years or following any incident or event that occurs which indicates that the pharmacy is not running safely and effectively
- identify the responsible pharmacist who reviewed the procedures
- identify which procedures are currently in place
- identify which procedures were previously in place

4.6 Make a temporary amendment to pharmacy procedures if the circumstances in the pharmacy change and in your professional opinion it is necessary to change the way in which the pharmacy normally operates

4.7 Ensure there is an audit trail to identify:

- which procedures are currently in place
- which procedures were previously in place
- the responsible pharmacist who amended the procedure, and
- the date on which the amendment was made,

if you make a temporary amendment to the pharmacy procedures

ABSENCE

The responsible pharmacist may be absent for up to a maximum period of two hours during the pharmacy's business hours between midnight and midnight. If there is more than one responsible pharmacist in charge of the registered pharmacy during the pharmacy's business hours, the total period of absence for all the responsible pharmacists concerned must not exceed two hours.

Only certain operational activities (see Appendix A) may be undertaken in the pharmacy if the responsible pharmacist in charge of the registered pharmacy is absent.

IF YOU ARE ABSENT YOU MUST:

5.1 Remain contactable with the pharmacy staff where this is reasonably practical and be able to return with reasonable promptness, where in your opinion this is necessary to secure the safe and effective running of the pharmacy

5.2 Arrange for another pharmacist to be available and contactable to provide advice to your pharmacy staff for any period of absence where it is not reasonably practicable to remain contactable and return with reasonable promptness

APPENDIX A – Examples of operational activities and the level of supervision required

A1 Activities which require a responsible pharmacist to be in charge of the premises (they may be absent for up to two hours per day), and need to take place under the supervision of a pharmacist and the supervising pharmacist will need to be physically present at the premises. This is not an exhaustive list.

ACTIVITY	UNDERPINNING LEGISLATION	OTHER REGULATORY CONSIDERATIONS
PROFESSIONAL CHECK (CLINICAL AND LEGAL CHECK) OF A PRESCRIPTION	The professional check is not required under the Medicines Act 1968. The responsible pharmacist / superintendent responsibilities covered by Sections 70, 71, 72 and 72A of the Medicines Act 1968	The check is required under NHS pharmaceutical services legislation
SALE/SUPPLY OF PHARMACY MEDICINES	Sections 52, 70, 71, 72 and 72A of the Medicines Act 1968	'Supervision' in this context requires physical presence and a pharmacist being able to advise and intervene
SALE/SUPPLY OF PRESCRIPTION-ONLY MEDICINES (E.G. HANDING DISPENSED MEDICINES OVER TO A PATIENT, PATIENT REPRESENTATIVE OR A DELIVERY PERSON)	Sections 52, 58, 70, 71, 72 and 72A of the Medicines Act 1968	'Supervision' in this context requires physical presence and a pharmacist being able to advise and intervene
SUPPLY OF MEDICINES UNDER A PATIENT GROUP DIRECTION	Sections 52, 58, 70, 71, 72 and 72A of the Medicines Act 1968. Articles 12A-12E of the Prescription Only Medicines (Human Use) Order 1997	'Supervision' in this context requires physical presence and a pharmacist being able to advise and intervene
WHOLESALE OF MEDICINES	Section 10(7) of the Medicines Act 1968	'Supervision' in this context requires physical presence and a pharmacist being able to advise and intervene
EMERGENCY SUPPLY OF A MEDICINE(S) AT THE REQUEST OF A PATIENT OR HEALTHCARE PROFESSIONAL	Sections 52, 58, 70, 71, 72 and 72A of the Medicines Act 1968. Article 8 of the Prescription Only Medicines (Human Use) Order 1997	'Supervision' in this context requires physical presence and a pharmacist being able to advise and intervene

RPS note: the Medicines Act 1968 is expected to have been consolidated with the bulk of medicines legislation sitting within the expected Human Medicines Regulations 2012

A2 Activities which require a responsible pharmacist to be in charge of the premises (they may be absent for up to two hours per day) and take place under the supervision of a pharmacist but who may not need to be physically present at the premises. This is not an exhaustive list.

ACTIVITY	UNDERPINNING LEGISLATION	OTHER REGULATORY CONSIDERATIONS
THE ASSEMBLY PROCESS (INCLUDING ASSEMBLY OF MONITORED DOSAGE SYSTEMS): ■ Generating a dispensing label ■ Taking medicines off the dispensary shelves ■ Assembly of the item (e.g. counting tablets) ■ Labelling of containers with the dispensing label ■ Accuracy checking	Section 10(1)(a) of the Medicines Act 1968	Supervision' in this context may not require the physical presence of a pharmacist. The level of supervision required of the suitably trained staff who undertake this work will depend on what is regarded as good practice within the pharmacy profession (see the note in this Appendix below)

A3 Activities which require a responsible pharmacist to be in charge of the premises (they may be absent for up to two hours) but does not require the supervision of a pharmacist. This is not an exhaustive list.

ACTIVITY	UNDERPINNING LEGISLATION	OTHER REGULATORY CONSIDERATIONS
SALE OF GENERAL SALES LIST MEDICINES	Sections 51, 70, 71, 72 and 72A of the Medicines Act 1968	Undertaken by suitable trained staff and operating within an agreed documented operating procedure

EXPLANATION OF 'ASSEMBLY'

The assembly of medicines against a prescription is controlled by Section 10 of the Medicines Act 1968.

In relating to a medicinal product 'assembly' is defined by the Medicines Act 1968 as:

enclosing the product (with or without other medicinal products of the same description) in a container which is labelled before the product is sold or supplied, or, where the product (with or without other medicinal products of the same description) is already enclosed in the container in which it is to be sold or supplied, labelling the container before the product is sold or supplied in it

Section 10 of the Medicines Act 1968 requires that the assembly process takes place under the 'supervision' of a pharmacist.

Supervision is not defined in the Act, and since the time the legislation was written the nature of assembly has changed in many instances. The introduction of patient packs has reduced the need to pack down or break bulk and the act of assembly often involves 'picking' the product rather than creating the final package or extemporaneously preparing medicines. The skills and competencies of staff undertaking dispensing activities have been developed and there is more emphasis of making full use of support staff releasing time for the pharmacist to provide a wider range of services. However, the legal definition remains the same.

The courts have considered the issue of the nature of 'supervision' required for the purposes of sale or supply of medicines and have concluded that, where supervision by a pharmacist is required, the actual transaction cannot take place without the physical presence of a pharmacist who is able to advise and intervene, even though s/he will not need to carry out the transaction themselves. However, the level of supervision required for assembly activities is less clear, and so for these activities, reference has to be made to more general case law of what 'supervision' means in the context of professional supervision.

The general position (derived from the Court of Appeal's judgment in Summers v Congreve Horner & Co [1992]

2 EGLR 152) is that supervision, in the context of professional supervision, means the degree of supervision required by what is regarded as good practice within the profession, having regard to the qualifications and experience of the person being supervised, but actual physical presence may not be necessary.

Applying that to the present context, it means that if the pharmacist responsible for supervising assembly of a medicinal product is absent, pharmacy support staff may continue to carry out activities which are considered to be "assembling" activities for the purposes of the definition set out above, without breaching the legislation, provided it is recognised good practice within the pharmacy profession that they be allowed to do so. The Royal Pharmaceutical Society publishes good practice guidance, but it is important to emphasise that no single solution fits all circumstances. What may be good practice for one type of assembling activity may not be good practice for other types of assembling activities, and all such activities must be "supervised" at an appropriate level.

It is also important to emphasise that this does not affect the position that the supply of assembled medicines against a prescription is prohibited unless the pharmacist is physically present in the registered pharmacy and in a position to advise and intervene. However, 'supervision' is not a 'one size fits all circumstances' legal concept, and the courts have recognised this.

APPENDIX B – The notice

The information that must be included on the notice is:

B1 Your name

B2 Your registration number

B3 That you are the responsible pharmacist in charge of that registered pharmacy premises

APPENDIX C – The pharmacy record

The details that must be recorded in the pharmacy record are:

C1 The responsible pharmacist's name

C2 The responsible pharmacist's registration number

C3 The date and time at which the responsible pharmacist became the responsible pharmacist

C4 The date and time at which the responsible pharmacist ceased to be the responsible pharmacist

C5 In relation to any absence of the responsible pharmacist from the registered pharmacy premises:

- the date of the absence
- the time at which the absence commenced
- the time at which the responsible pharmacist returned to the registered pharmacy premises

APPENDIX D – Pharmacy procedures

The matters which must be covered by pharmacy procedures are:

D1 The arrangements to secure that medicinal products are:

- ordered
- stored
- prepared
- sold by retail
- supplied in circumstances corresponding to retail sale
- delivered outside the pharmacy
- disposed of in a safe and effective manner

D2 The circumstances in which a member of pharmacy staff who is not a pharmacist may give advice about medicinal products

D3 The identification of members of pharmacy staff who are, in the view of the responsible pharmacist, competent to perform certain tasks relating to the pharmacy business

D4 The keeping of records about the arrangements mentioned in paragraph D1

D5 The arrangements which are to apply during the absence of the responsible pharmacist from the premises

D6 The steps to be taken when there is a change of responsible pharmacist at the premises

D7 The procedure which is to be followed if a complaint is made about the pharmacy business

D8 The procedure which is to be followed if an incident occurs which may indicate that the pharmacy business is not running in a safe and effective manner

D9 The manner in which changes to the pharmacy procedures are to be notified to pharmacy staff.

RPS Support note – by the time of publication of MEP 36 the consolidation and review of the Medicines Act is expected and many sections will be superseded by the Human Medicines Regulations 2012.

APPENDIX 11: GPhC GUIDANCE ON RESPONDING TO COMPLAINTS AND CONCERNS

The General Pharmaceutical Council is the regulator for pharmacists, pharmacy technicians and registered pharmacy premises in England, Scotland and Wales.

This document provides guidance on dealing with complaints and concerns raised by patients, the public and other healthcare professionals.

We are providing this guidance to assist pharmacy professionals on how to best meet the responsibilities that a pharmacy owner or pharmacy professional has in relation to handling and managing complaints and concerns.

As dispensing errors are frequently the basis for complaints, we will also provide guidance on:

- How to minimise the risk of a dispensing error occurring
- What to do in the event of a dispensing error
- How to review dispensing errors

This Guidance Note has been published by the Standards Advisory Team. If you have questions about its content, please contact us on 020 3365 3640 or via email at standards@pharmacyregulation.org.

This Guidance Note will next be reviewed in October 2011

INTRODUCTION

The standards of conduct, ethics and performance must be followed by pharmacists and registered pharmacy technicians. Principle 1 of these standards is to "make patients your first concern". A requirement under this principle is to "organise regular reviews, audits and risk assessments to protect patient and public safety and to improve your professional service".

The standards also require you to have standard operating procedures (SOPs) in place which must be followed at all times.

The standards for pharmacy owners and superintendent pharmacists of retail pharmacy businesses require pharmacy owners and superintendent pharmacists

to ensure the safe and effective running of the pharmacy. To allow this there must be appropriate policies, procedures and records in place that are maintained and reviewed regularly. There must also be an appropriate mechanism in place to respond to and investigate all complaints and concerns raised.

The standards referred to above can be found at **www.pharmacyregulation.org.**

WHY COMPLAINTS ARISE

There are numerous reasons for why a complaint or concern may arise. The majority of complaints or concerns are due to:

- Human error
- System failure, for example when a pharmacy doesn't have adequate SOPs in place
- How a complaint or concern is handled in the pharmacy

The way in which a complaint or concern is handled in the pharmacy can determine whether or not it is then referred to an independent body such as the General Pharmaceutical Council (GPhC) or the primary care organisation (PCO).

HOW TO DEAL WITH A COMPLAINT OR CONCERN THAT HAS BEEN RAISED

When something goes wrong or someone reports a concern to you, you should make sure you deal with it appropriately.

There should be an effective complaints procedure where you work and you must follow it at all times.

You should make a record of the complaint, concern or incident and the action taken. You should review your records and findings and audit them regularly.

DISPENSING ERRORS

The investigating committee considered 732 cases between April 2009 and March 2010. Approximately 32% of these cases concerned dispensing errors. The Disciplinary Committee considered 396 cases during the same period of which 15% concerned dispensing errors.

HOW TO MINIMISE THE RISK OF MAKING A DISPENSING ERROR

DISPENSARY LAYOUT:

- The dispensary should be organised to keep distractions to a minimum
- The atmosphere of the dispensary should encourage good concentration
- Alert staff to the dangers of stock being placed in the wrong location. Dispensary stock should only be put away by a competent member of staff
- Keep a segregated area of the dispensary workbench for the dispensing process
- Segregate prescriptions on the workbench to avoid patients receiving someone else's medicines. You may use baskets / trays if appropriate

DISPENSING PROCESS:

- Produce dispensing labels before any product is selected from the shelf
- Do not select stock using dispensing labels or patient medication records (PMR). Refer to the prescription when selecting stock for dispensing
- Dispense items from the prescription and not the generated label
- You should have systems in place to identify who was involved in the dispensing and checking process of each prescription item (e.g. dispensed by / checked by boxes)
- Two people should be involved in the dispensing process where this is possible. A second competent person should carry out an accuracy check and ideally should not have been involved in the assembly process
- If you are a pharmacist working alone, once you have assembled the medicines, try to create a short mental break between the assembly and final check to avoid carrying over any recollection of preconceived errors from the assembly process

- All accuracy checks should be made against the original prescription re-reading the prescription first
- Dispense balances of medication owed by reference only to the original prescription or a good quality copy. Do not rely solely on the information in the PMR or an owing note or label. This will prevent you making the same error that may have previously been made by another pharmacist

The National Patient Safety Agency (NPSA) (**www.npsa.nhs.uk**) has published a document entitled "A guide to the design of dispensed medicines", which looks at the key aspects of labelling and presentation of a dispensed medicine.

Another publication, entitled "A guide to the design of dispensing environments", provides guidance on how the design of a dispensary can improve patient safety. Whilst the physical design of the dispensary can inevitably improve the working environment and therefore patient safety other things should also be considered. For example, the workflow and how the dispensary area is utilised can improve the efficiency and improve safety.

WHAT TO DO IN THE EVENT OF A DISPENSING ERROR

Pharmacists should carry out a root cause analysis in the event of a patient safety incident. This is a retrospective technique for looking for the underlying causes of a patient safety incident, behind the immediate and obvious cause. For example, one individual's human error might be the immediate cause, but several factors could have contributed to the error such as fatigue, an inadequate checking system or poor standard operating procedures.

The NPSA is promoting root cause analysis and is encouraging organisations to identify the circumstances in which it should be used. This should take into account the severity of the incident and the scope for learning from it. Further information on root cause analysis can be found on the NPSA website at **www.npsa.nhs.uk**.

You may wish to consider all the points below when dealing with an error or handling a complaint. In addition, locum pharmacists may also wish to keep their own records in case they are contacted later.

When the patient first comes in or indicates that there has been an error:

■ **ESTABLISH IF THE PATIENT HAS TAKEN ANY OF THE INCORRECT MEDICINE**

If the patient has taken any of the incorrect medicine, establish whether the patient has been harmed. If they have been harmed, provide the complainant and the patient's GP with the advice they need immediately. Contact the local drug information centre, if appropriate, for advice on the possible effects on the patient (giving details of concurrent medication). Where no harm appears to have been caused, the GP should still be informed.

■ **ASK TO INSPECT THE INCORRECT MEDICINE**

Make it clear that you do not wish to retain the medication, and that inspecting the medicine can give valuable clues about what went wrong. If the patient does not want to hand the medicine over to you, suggest that they retain it until they can hand it over to an appropriate representative of the GPhC or their local PCO. Incorrect medicines should not routinely be posted to these organisations.

If the patient does hand over and leave the incorrect medication with you retain it and keep it segregated from stock and other medicines to be supplied to patients.

Never dispose of any medicine unless the patient has given consent. Before doing so it should be retained carefully, for a reasonable period, in case of further developments.

■ **APOLOGISE**

In the case of a dispensing error, an apology should not be confused with an admission of liability.

■ **NEVER TRY TO MINIMISE THE SERIOUSNESS OF AN ERROR**

A balance must be struck that reassures the patient, if no harm is likely, but without suggesting that the error is insignificant.

■ **MAKE A SUPPLY OF THE CORRECT MEDICINE ORDERED ON THE PRESCRIPTION, IF APPROPRIATE**

You can lawfully make a supply of the correct medicine as this was authorised on the original prescription, even in the case of a controlled drug. Where the patient has not taken any of the incorrect medication it is your professional judgment about whether the patient's GP needs to be informed.

■ **ESTABLISH THEIR EXPECTATIONS**

It is important to establish what the complainant would like you to do about their complaint.

■ **PROVIDE DETAILS OF HOW TO COMPLAIN TO AN 'OFFICIAL BODY' IF REQUESTED**

Supply the complainant with the name and address of the Fitness to Practise Department of the GPhC if the complainant feels that the only way forward is to complain to an 'official body'. Explain that a Professional Standards Inspector from the GPhC may visit the pharmacy to undertake a review. You may also provide the details of the PCO so that the matter can be dealt with under the NHS complaints procedure.

■ **TRY AND ESTABLISH WHAT HAPPENED AND WHAT WENT WRONG**

You may need to make your own inquiries into any possible causes of the alleged error for preventative purposes unless it is clear from the facts known to you, how the error is likely to have occurred. You may need to speak to the person who presented or collected the prescription about the prevailing conditions in the pharmacy. Contact the complainant and inform them of your findings.

■ **FOLLOW COMPANY PROCEDURES / SOPS FOR REPORTING ERRORS OR COMPLAINTS**

Where you are an employee pharmacist, you should follow the procedures laid down by your employer/ Superintendent for who you should notify in the event of a dispensing error. If you are working within a company, you may have to report any errors to your line manager and/or a Superintendent office. You must follow company procedures for such reporting and may wish to consult the superintendent pharmacist and other line managers for advice.

■ **RECORD, REVIEW AND LEARN FROM ERRORS MADE**

See section on reviewing errors.

■ **NOTIFY THE PHARMACIST WHO WAS ON DUTY AT THE TIME, IF IT WAS NOT YOU**

You may use the Responsible Pharmacist record to ascertain who was on duty at the time.

- **INFORM YOUR PROFESSIONAL INDEMNITY INSURANCE PROVIDER**

  In all cases of dispensing errors, the over-riding responsibility is for the health and well-being of the patient. Whilst keeping this in mind, you should inform your professional indemnity insurers as soon as possible, in case a claim is later made against you.

REVIEWING ERRORS

Make a written record of your findings when you carry out your review to establish what went wrong. You can record your findings using the mnemonic "CHAPS" to cover the various areas of the supply. CHAPS covers the following points:

C CONDITIONS IN THE PHARMACY AT THE TIME

This can be established from the:

- Complainant
- Records – records would help to identify the name of the responsible pharmacist and whether they had been working without a break
- Computer – computer records may help to identify the number of prescriptions dispensed that day and the exact time the prescription was dispensed

Interestingly most errors do not occur during busy periods of dispensing.

You may wish to review the layout of the dispensary and the availability of bench space. You may use baskets or similar to hold dispensed items before checking and handing to the patient with counselling. It has been reported that pharmacists who use this type of system help prevent medicines being crossed from one patient to another, and also to keep the bench space tidy.

H HEALTH OF THE PHARMACIST AND OTHER MEMBERS OF THE TEAM

Was the pharmacist or other person(s) involved in the dispensing process ill at the time?

A ASSISTANCE

Was the pharmacist working alone or was s/he assisted? Identify the person who assisted. Make a judgment about the qualifications and competence of the assistant.

P PRESCRIPTION SHOULD BE RECOVERED FROM THE FILE OR GET A COPY OF IT FROM THE RELEVANT PRESCRIPTION PRICING AUTHORITY

- Was the error caused by the legibility of the prescription?
- Was the prescription hand written or computer generated?
- Check endorsements for what was supplied

S SYSTEMS USED FOR DISPENSING AND CHECKING MUST BE REVIEWED

Depending upon whether the pharmacist was working alone or with someone assisting, this covers every part of the dispensing process. The type of error may direct your attention to one area of dispensing practice.

Usually errors fall into categories:

- Misreading the prescription
- Incorrect picking of the medicines
- Transposing the label or labelling the medicine incorrectly
- Giving the wrong prescription to the wrong patient (for example, where the error involves placing the medicine in the wrong bag or where the patient's address is not checked properly when handing out the dispensed medicine)
- Selection of the wrong strength (or wrong preparation) from the PMRs when using the repeats facility, then checking the stock against the label, not the original prescription
- Incorrect compounding
- Supplying contaminated or out-of-date stock
- Dispensing against an incorrectly written owing slip, rather than the prescription

Whatever weaknesses there are in the system, the final accuracy check must overcome them. It is most important to review these critically.

The mnemonic "HELP" can be used when making the final check on the dispensed medicine, to ensure that all the necessary checks have been made. HELP stands for the following:

H "HOW MUCH" HAS BEEN DISPENSED

Open all unsealed cartons and sealed cartons, if appropriate, to check that the contents are correct and match the quantity requested on the prescription. Check that the correct patient information leaflet has been included.

E "EXPIRY DATE" CHECK

Ensure this is sufficient to cover the treatment period.

L "LABEL" CHECK

Check the patient's name, product name, form, strength and dose are the same as on the prescription. Check that the correct and appropriate warning(s) are included on the label.

P "PRODUCT" CHECK

Check that the correct medication and strength which has been requested on the prescription has been supplied.

Handing out of dispensed medicines must be carried out by trained staff. To avoid handing medicines to the wrong person, prescription receipts may provide useful safeguards, although even these are not foolproof. The person collecting the dispensed medicine should be asked for the address or date of birth of the patient, which should be checked against the prescription.

When reviewing dispensing errors which have resulted in a serious patient safety incident, the NPSA incident decision tree helps to identify why individuals acted in a certain way, and this may be a very useful tool for pharmacists, managers and organisations to consider using. Information on the incident decision tree can be found at **www.npsa.nhs.uk.**

INDEX